Dr. Abdullah has written the most accurate and practical book on skincare today. His clear and easy-to-understand principles and applications brilliantly bridge the gap between the science of skin and clinical skincare."
—STEVEN S. CARP, MD, AMERICAN BOARD OF PLASTIC SURGERY—CERTIFIED
 SURGEON AT CARP COSMETIC SURGERY CENTER

For the past three decades, I've helped launch several skincare lines that turned into global brands, so I thought I knew a lot about the subject. Dr. Abdullah's book made me realize that many commonly held beliefs about skin "science"— on topics such as collagen, elastin, oxygen, moisturizers, and exfoliation—are all *wrong*! His commonsense approach clears up these misconceptions and sets readers on a much simpler and more affordable path to younger-looking skin."
—JEFFERY GODDARD, FOUNDER AND CEO OF TVA MEDIA GROUP

Dr. Abdullah has provided a great service by getting back to the basics of skincare The concepts of the science behind modern skincare are discussed with great clarity. This book is a must-read for everyone who wants to look great and improve the quality and appearance of their skin."
—LOUIS L. STROCK, MD, FACS, AMERICAN BOARD OF PLASTIC SURGERY—
 CERTIFIED SURGEON

This is a wonderful book, with a strong scientific base yet written in terms that can be understood without a medical background. It serves as a great reference for both physicians and patients alike."
—LINDA G. PHILLIPS, MD, TRUMAN G. BLOCKER JR., MD, DISTINGUISHED
 PROFESSOR AND CHIEF, DIVISION OF PLASTIC SURGERY, AT UNIVERSITY OF
 TEXAS MEDICAL BRANCH AT GALVESTON

'*Simple Skincare, Beautiful Skin* will forever change the way consumers view skincare companies and skincare products. Dr. Abdullah provides an honest, practical approach to skincare that, when put into practice, will save consumers the cost and frustration of buying useless products. A must-read for consumers and the perfect reference for skincare professionals!"
—HEATHER FOWLER, LICENSED ESTHETICIAN AND OWNER AT RENEW SKIN THERAPY

SIMPLE SKINCARE, BEAUTIFUL SKIN

A BACK-TO-BASICS APPROACH

AHMED ABDULLAH MD, FACS, FICS

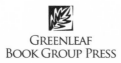

GREENLEAF
BOOK GROUP PRESS

This book is intended as a reference volume only, not as a medical manual. The information given here is designed to help you make informed decisions about your health. It is not intended as a substitute for any treatment that may have been prescribed by your doctor. If you suspect that you have a medical problem, you should seek competent medical help. You should not begin a new health regimen without first consulting a medical professional.

Published by Greenleaf Book Group Press
Austin, Texas
www.gbgpress.com

Distributed by Greenleaf Book Group LLC

For ordering information or special discounts for bulk purchases, please contact Greenleaf Book Group LLC at PO Box 91869, Austin, TX 78709, 512.891.6100.

Design and composition by Greenleaf Book Group LLC
Cover design by Greenleaf Book Group LLC
Cover photo ©iStockphoto.com/gruizza
Author photo by Harley Danielson

Publisher's Cataloging-In-Publication Data
(Prepared by The Donohue Group, Inc.)
Abdullah, Ahmed, 1958-
    Simple skincare, beautiful skin : a back-to-basics approach / Ahmed Abdullah. ~ 1st ed.
    p. : ill. ; cm.
    Issued also as an ebook.
    Includes bibliographical references.
    ISBN: 978-1-60832-383-8

    1. Skin~Care and hygiene. 2. Beauty, Personal. I. Title. II. Title: Simple skin care, beautiful skin
RL87 .A23 2012
646.7/26   2012937093

Part of the Tree Neutral® program, which offsets the number of trees consumed in the production and printing of this book by taking proactive steps, such as planting trees in direct proportion to the number of trees used: www.treeneutral.com

Printed in the United States of America on acid-free paper

12 13 14 15 16 17   10 9 8 7 6 5 4 3 2 1

First Edition

CONTENTS

ACKNOWLEDGMENTS

This book would not have been possible without the support and encouragement of my family, friends, and educators. Sincere thanks and appreciation are owed to many, including:

My wife Kay, who not only provides moral support at every step but was also an invaluable resource as I wrote this book. Along the way she put her medical background to use by offering pertinent advice and double-checking the science and facts I presented.

My sons Ali and Alex for being my shining lights and helping me find my way in life.

My parents and sisters, Anjum and Anees, for consistently supporting my goals and ambitions ever since I was a child. I must especially recognize my father's unending belief in me. It was his encouragement that led me to become a physician.

My teachers and mentors throughout my academic career. I want to make special mention of the following individuals who made a significant impact on my evolution as a scientist and physician to date: Mrs. Mujahid and Mr. Khalilullah from Karachi Grammar School, who taught me biology and helped me recognize my zeal for the subject, while pointing me toward my future as a scientist; Dr. David Herndon, Dr. Marty Robson, and Dr. John Heggers, for challenging me always and inculcating in me a love for research and discovery. I am especially grateful to Dr. Robson for teaching me about aloe vera and its amazing properties. Without that, none of this would have been possible.

PREFACE

There is little doubt that skincare has become downright confusing. Just look in your medicine cabinet and you'll see what I mean. If you're like most people, you'll find a dizzying array of cleansers, toners, moisturizers, serums, exfoliants, eye creams, scrubs, masks, wrinkle creams, brightening gels, pore minimizers, fade creams, and more. Look a bit closer and you'll find product labeling that touts new ingredients sure to erase your skin concerns. But are you satisfied? I assume you wouldn't be reading this book if you were.

Given that the needs of our skin are relatively simple, it's hard to believe that skincare ever got so complicated. But considering the dollars the industry spends on marketing, it's no wonder. Advertising campaigns have created an overwhelmed consumer who spends far more money than they should in an attempt to improve their skin.

So why this book? First, let me tell you what it is not. It won't give you a magic solution for taking years off your face. I firmly believe the last thing people need is yet another new beauty regimen that delivers disappointing results. Rather, this book is about undoing everything you've learned about skincare and paring down your knowledge to the vital facts, while giving you scientific and sound solutions to ensuring optimal skin health. Essentially, it's about going back to basics—a concept that is easily lost in this industry. While some of the information included here you've undoubtedly heard before, there's much that I'm certain will be new. Regardless, this book is intended as a compendium of the proven steps that, if followed faithfully, will most assuredly result in improved skin health and, thus, aesthetics.

Since becoming a plastic and cosmetic surgeon nearly twenty years ago, I've learned that healthy skin does more than simply enhance the natural beauty of an individual; it also improves their confidence and overall happiness. With this book as a guide, I'm determined to help you do both.

Ahmed Abdullah, MD, FACS, FICS

RECONSIDER WHAT YOU KNOW ABOUT SKINCARE; IT MAY BE ALL WRONG

For centuries, humans have been searching for the exact formulation of ingredients that will erase the signs of aging from their faces. Today, that pursuit has hit record proportions, with Americans spending nearly $1.6 billion on anti-aging skincare products alone.[1] Yet, ask these individuals if they're happy with the results they're getting from these products and you're certain to get a lukewarm response. In fact, of those who use anti-aging products, only 3 percent claim to have used them because they found them effective.[2]

This statistic comes as no surprise to me. Throughout my nearly twenty years in practice as a plastic and cosmetic surgeon, countless patients—both women and men—have told me stories of spending hundreds and even thousands of dollars on products that promised to deliver a youthful appearance but did little more than smell good. Despite this, the number one question I'm asked remains, "What product do you recommend I use to remove wrinkles?" As consumers, we continue to hold out hope that the fountain of youth really can be found in a jar.

Motivated by a consumer willingness to spend dollar after dollar on skincare that promises to turn back the hands of time, cosmetic companies have sent their product development teams into overdrive. The result: Thousands of products are launched each year featuring "revolutionary" new ingredients or "miracle" formulations and accompanied by marketing campaigns that feature scientific claims and flawless models. Who can blame people for being convinced?

When my patients tell me about the disappointing products they've used, they inevitably defend their purchase by referring to the science that backed the products' claims. You know what they're talking about: "clinically proven to reduce wrinkles in seven days," or "after four weeks, 90 percent reported that fine lines had faded away." While many companies do cite justifiable, independent research to back product ingredients, of concern are the organizations that tout biased findings. We need to be certain that the claims are founded on "good science" and are, thus, valid.

COMMON MYTHS

While commonly accepted myths are prevalent in many consumer industries, they run particularly rampant in the skincare category. Given the emotion that accompanies the desire to improve one's appearance, marketers have been able to convince consumers of many factors that, at face value, don't make much sense. It's as though the trendy product design and incredible before and after photos erode one's better judgment.

Some of my favorite skincare myths are outlined below. You'll also find the facts that debunk them.

PRODUCTS CONTAINING COLLAGEN AND/ OR ELASTIN CAN REJUVENATE SKIN CELLS.

Countless advertisements in recent years exclaim a product's use of collagen and/or elastin. These are major structural proteins in our skin that are often advertised to have magical qualities when applied topically. However, the reality is that, when added to a product, collagen or elastin has <u>absolutely no benefit</u> to the skin whatsoever. At most, they may make the product consistency "feel" more silky and smooth.

Here's why:

Collagen and elastin are proteins found in our skin and in that of all animals. These proteins comprise the structure of the dermal layer of the skin. However, collagen and elastin cannot be absorbed into the skin because their moleculer size is too large, a step that would be essential if they were to do any good whatsoever. What's more, if you take them out of a human or animal source, the proteins are dead. Therefore, even if the skin could absorb them, they're completely inactive and would not provide any benefit. The only collagen or elastin our bodies can use is that created by our own cells and tissues. That from another human or animal source is completely useless.

Say for a moment, however, that collagen and elastin did have some beneficial properties when applied topically to the skin. It would then be important to note the type of collagen or elastin that is used. Most collagen and elastin found on ingredient lists is referred to as "soluble collagen" or "hydrolyzed elastin." This means the manufacturer has actually cut the molecule into tiny pieces. Therefore, even if they were beneficial, you aren't getting true collagen or elastin in these products—only pieces of these proteins.

The only benefit of using collagen and elastin in skincare products is the improvement it brings to the consistency of the product. In other words, they make the product feel nice on the skin.

PRODUCTS CONTAINING OXYGEN ENSURE YOUTHFUL-LOOKING SKIN.

Given that oxygen is essential to life, its usage on our skin must be beneficial, right? Wrong.

Simply put, we need approximately 23% oxygen in the air we breathe to live. Anything more than that may be converted into O_3, otherwise known as oxidants or free radicals. This fact alone demonstrates that oxygen in skincare products isn't beneficial. However, let's go a step further and look at a few additional realities. First, humans cannot absorb oxygen through the skin; it is only absorbed through the lungs. From an evolutionary standpoint, if our skin could absorb oxygen, our lungs wouldn't have developed. Second—and here's the real catch—oxygen cannot even be put into a skincare product because it's a gas. It simply won't mix with the product's other added ingredients. Even if it could be contained in a product formulation, it would release into the atmosphere rather than penetrate the skin when applied, due to its gaseous state. Therefore, any marketing that claims a product contains pure oxygen is little more than false advertising.

FACIAL SKIN REQUIRES MULTIPLE MOISTURIZERS.

It is a common misconception that skin needs numerous, separate moisturizers for different areas of the face. The skin does need a good moisturizer, the type of which is dependent upon skin type. For instance, oily skin requires a moisturizer with less oil-based humectants, while very dry skin needs a moisturizer with heavier humectants. However, there is no absolute need to buy separate moisturizers for different parts of your face.

SEPARATE EYE CREAM IS ESSENTIAL.

The skin around the eyes is thinner and has fewer oil glands. Therefore, it does require extra care. However, use of a hydrating moisturizer works just fine if carefully applied around the eyes. Skin is skin, so what works on the rest of your face works in this area, as well.

If trying, specifically, to improve the appearance of fine lines, puffiness, and dark circles, then a separate eye product such as a serum or gel-formulated product with extra emollients may be considered.

THE CONCEPT OF "GENTLE EXFOLIATION."

There is no such thing as "gentle exfoliation." By its nature, exfoliation requires force or strong acid to remove dead and damaged skin cells. Only by being aggressive with exfoliation will it give the desired effect of collagen stimulation and dermal rejuvenation. Although rubbing the skin with "granules" or "microspheres" may give a temporary polished feel to the skin, it will not provide the necessary force to slough dead skin cells and boost collagen production.

PRODUCTS THAT ARE "DERMATOLOGIST RECOMMENDED" OR "DERMATOLOGIST TESTED" ARE PROVEN TO WORK.

Phrases like "dermatologist recommended" or "dermatologist tested" simply mean that as few as one dermatologist has tried the product or used it on a patient with no negative results. It is in no way valid proof of a product's performance.

MEN AND WOMEN REQUIRE DIFFERENT SKINCARE PRODUCTS.

In recent years, there has been an increase in the number of skincare products formulated specifically for men. Remember the tenant that "skin is skin?" The same rule applies here. Of course, *individuals* have different concerns and, thus, require differing approaches to skincare. But these differences cannot simply be divided down gender lines.

Given the recent growth of the male personal care market, it's no wonder that companies are putting out skincare lines targeted specifically to this audience. However, the only difference between these products and other skincare lines is the fragrance and the look of the bottles. After all, few men want a "cute" bottle on their bathroom shelf!

EXPENSIVE SKINCARE PRODUCTS FROM ESTABLISHED BRANDS ARE THE MOST EFFECTIVE.

This is exactly what the marketers of these brands want you to think. In reality, this statement is far from true. These brands, most of which invest far more in marketing than in product research and development, gain their "well known" reputation through aggressive advertising campaigns.

WATER-BASED SKINCARE PRODUCTS KEEP YOUR SKIN HYDRATED.

This is, in my opinion, one of the biggest myths within the skincare industry. Water-based skincare products don't hydrate because the skin cannot absorb water. The presence of water simply dilutes the active ingredients that *are* contained within the product.

Motivated by my patients' obvious frustration and confusion about skincare, in 1996 I embarked on a yearlong quest to find the best skincare line. I wanted to give my patients a strong recommendation when they asked what products to use pre- and post-procedure and for ongoing maintenance of their skin.

My background certainly was helpful in this endeavor. A significant part of my surgical training was spent working with burns and exploring elements that impact wound healing. In fact, I conducted research on the growth factors involved in skin repair at a cellular level. Additionally, I was aided by an expert knowledge of organic chemistry, biology, and pharmacology.

Given that my surgical mentor, Dr. Martin Robson, past chair of the American Board of Plastic Surgery, was recognized worldwide for his research on the benefits of aloe in healing, I was influenced to utilize high-grade aloe in my surgical practice. After all, I saw firsthand how the application of aloe to skin flaps in surgery has a remarkable ability to prevent tissue damage and accelerate healing. Robson's work encouraged me to pursue my own research into potential applications for aloe within a clinical environment and, thus, I've authored numerous studies proving its benefits in conditions ranging from frostbite and burns to diabetes. These experiences, including the results I've seen in my own practice, have continually convinced me that aloe vera is a powerhouse ingredient for use in sensible skincare. Aloe vera has immense and manifold benefits to the skin, and its effectiveness has been proven not only in the laboratory but in human studies, as well. Because of this, I became particularly interested in developing a line of skincare products that could properly use aloe's valuable properties.

The research project was eye opening, at minimum. I was surprised to find that nearly every skincare brand I encountered—whether physician-dispensed or over-the-counter, drugstore or department store, organic or conventional—utilized a base of water. When aloe was utilized, it was in minute quantities and of inadequate quality to generate results. I began to realize that product formulations were often more marketing than science. Most formulations I reviewed had little hope of ever accomplishing the results for which they were intended, and I was left feeling disenchanted. In good faith, I couldn't recommend any single brand to my patients. What's more, I realized it was essential that consumers become educated about the basic needs of their skin to prevent the continued frustration they were encountering. With that, I've spent the past ten years providing this knowledge to each of my patients, and it's that knowledge that I share with you.

While I now formulate skincare products utilizing a base of pharmaceutical-grade aloe and ingredients proven by unbiased science to benefit the skin, it is important I note that, beyond my brand, many good skincare products do exist. However, rather than blindly trusting a single brand, buying a bundled regimen, or placing hope in a product that makes big promises, it's important to review each formulation independently to determine if it will work for your skin. Through the pages of this book, I will give you the skills you need to become an empowered consumer of skincare.

FACING THE FACTS

The simple truth is that the aging process cannot be reversed, and, thus, it's important that consumers are realistic about the results they'll achieve by using a skincare formulation. While there are certainly methods available to mask one's age (I should know; I've made a career of it), they do not come from a bottle. However, the importance of *healthy* skin cannot be underestimated for what it can do to improve the aesthetics of the skin. Advanced formulations are, indeed, capable of greatly improving characteristics associated with poor skin health, such as rough texture and fine lines dramatized by a lack of exfoliation, and diminishment of the skin's ability to produce collagen and elastin. You see, healthy skin is beautiful skin. And skincare products can help your skin reach its peak condition.

In the chapters that follow, we're going to cover a lot of territory. But as we embark on this journey, there are several key facts I want you to keep in mind:

1. The most effective skincare regimen is one that is simple.
2. If a product sounds too good to be true, it probably is.
3. Maintaining an effective skincare regimen should not cost you a fortune.
4. There are no shortcuts on the path to beautiful skin. Getting there requires a commitment to healthy behaviors.
5. An advertisement should never be the tool by which you decide the skincare products you'll buy. By becoming educated, you empower yourself to objectively evaluate claims and select products that will meet the needs of your skin.

With that, let's get started.

2

THE BASICS OF SKIN SCIENCE

As the covering that surrounds us, skin is charged with the vital task of protecting internal organs from the dangerous elements of the world. It is our body's first line of defense and, thus, prevents the invasion of non-resident bacteria. It also regulates temperature and provides us with sensory information. Given its importance, our primary concern is to ensure its health. By maintaining healthy skin, we make certain it can perform its important functions, while bene-fitting from improved aesthetic characteristics, including smooth, soft texture; absence of blemishes; even coloring; small pore size; and overall radiance.

For an example of optimal skin health, one needs only to look at a baby. Infant skin is properly hydrated and free from damage, resulting in an ideal appearance. Of course, it isn't realistic for an adult to expect skin so flawless, but this model demonstrates what skin looks like when proper nutrition is provided to the body, and factors like excessive sun exposure or smoking have not been introduced. Unfortunately, some skin damage is a natural part of the body's aging process. Lines and wrinkles are inevitable and will increase with age. Thus, our goal must be to *optimize* skin health while having realistic expectations for what our skin should look like given our age, medical history, and past behaviors.

While a sound knowledge of skin biology and physiology is unnecessary to achieving optimal skin health, having a basic understanding of the composition of skin and the factors that impact it is certainly beneficial. Armed with this information, you will be better able to interpret the "science speak" found on skincare products and more objectively evaluate product claims. It also helps bring logic to the necessary steps involved in improving skin health.

SKIN COMPOSITION

Of course, there's more to the skin than that which you see on the surface. Human skin is comprised of three main layers—the epidermis, dermis, and hypodermis—each of which carries out a key role in protecting the body. To prevent disruption to the body's nutrients, skin is water-resistant. And to prevent fluid loss, it is semi-impermeable. These points are important when considering skincare product formulations and are ones we'll return to in a later chapter.

The skin is a complicated structure with numerous layers within the three main layers, each of which is specific in its function.

For the purposes of this discussion, let's review the three main layers:

EPIDERMIS

The epidermis is the visible, external section of the skin, mainly comprised of keratinocytes—cells that produce keratin, a protein that protects the skin. Five layers comprise the epidermis. At the bottom layer (the stratum basale), new cells are produced. These cells continuously migrate up through the layers of the epidermis, flattening as they go, until they reach the outermost layer (stratum corneum), which contains dead keratinocytes. The stratum corneum layer is shed every thirty days, approximately.

Depending on the area of the body, the epidermis may be extremely thin, as in eyelids, or thick, such as on the soles of the feet or palms of the hands.

DERMIS

The middle section, the dermis, acts as a factory for the skin. Here, proteins are made, including collagen, which provides skin strength, and elastin, which provides skin elasticity and structure. This layer also houses hair follicles, blood and lymph vessels, nerves, sweat glands, and sebaceous glands that produce an oily-like substance called sebum. It is in this skin layer that wrinkles are formed.

HYPODERMIS

The innermost section of skin, and the thickest of the three, is the hypodermis. This layer is comprised mainly of adipose tissue (the body's fat stores). Additionally, the hypodermis contains connective tissue, large nerves, and blood vessels.

Of these layers, the epidermis is the primary target of most skincare products, as their ability is generally limited to the skin's surface. However, some skincare formulations have the capacity to affect the operations of the dermis layer, and, more specifically, the production of collagen and elastin. Behaviors such as proper nutrition, hydration, good oxygenation, and the relative absence of stress positively impact the dermis layer, the skin's manufacturing site. This optimal skin health can only be achieved when good internal and external practices are employed simultaneously.

SKIN DAMAGE

When skin health is compromised, there's simply no way to deny it. Within a short span of time, skin that has been damaged or mistreated begins to show symptoms, such as a feeling of tightness or dryness; pigmentation changes, including brown or red spots and melasma (darkened skin on sun-exposed areas); uneven and rough texture; acne; enlarged pore size; general redness; visibility of abnormal capillaries; and, yes, wrinkles.

Skin damage is typically grouped into four categories: *environmental, chronological, medical,* and *hereditary.* However, because skin is the only organ in the body that gets damaged not only from the exterior but also from the interior, I suggest a fifth category of *nutrition.* A body that suffers from an unbalanced diet or improper hydration will indeed show signs of damage. (We'll explore the topic of nutrition and your skin in chapter 3.)

ENVIRONMENTAL

As the body's suit of armor against the outside world, skin is affected by the environmental conditions it encounters. If proper precautions are not taken to protect it from these environmental factors, skin health is impacted, resulting in so many of the aesthetic symptoms outlined earlier. Therefore, environmental skin damage differs significantly from person to person, dependent upon their behaviors.

Among the most prevalent environmental factors are pollution, which robs our skin of vitamin E and causes skin dehydration; smoking, which depletes collagen and thins the skin, encourages the formation of lines and wrinkles, and leaves the skin with a slight grey pigmentation; and the sun, which causes pigment changes, depletion of collagen levels, broken capillaries, skin lesions, and, of course, the potential for skin cancer. This environmental skin damage is mostly related to an increase in free radicals in aging skin tissue. Factors such as UV light and the presence of toxins encourage the production of free radicals.

CHRONOLOGICAL

Aging is generally the main cause of skin damage. A natural aspect of human life, it is simply inevitable. As the skin begins showing signs of aging—often around the age of twenty-five—one of the first areas to demonstrate damage is the periphery of the eye. Here, the development of dark circles, puffiness, and crow's feet may become apparent. The rate at which skin shows the signs of aging varies by individual and is simply due to genetics. Look at aging skin microscopically, and you see skin cells beginning to decay and the dermis thinning due to a loss of collagen.

When the skin is young, it is better equipped to deal with damaging factors, as repair mechanisms are at their peak. As such, signs of environmental damage and aging may not be clearly visible. With the advancement in age, however, these repair mechanisms begin to function less efficiently. Skin cells are not shed as easily, and the rate at which our skin cells renew is diminished significantly. Additionally, collagen and elastin levels begin to diminish. Thus, skin damage manifests itself in the form of wrinkles, age spots, changes in pore size, sagging skin, and a general rough texture. If the skin fails to receive appropriate and effective treatment during this period, the damage worsens. This results in aged, leathery skin with uneven texture.

MEDICAL

The skin may be affected by various medical conditions, infections, and even the prescription drugs used to treat them. Additionally, trauma may cause significant damage to the skin. Hormone changes with aging also contribute heavily to skin degeneration.

HEREDITY

Some skin damage may be out of our control due to hereditary conditions and genetic disorders. For example, some individuals are predisposed to psoriasis, eczema, or keratosis pilaris, which may have a lasting impact on the skin.

SOLUTIONS FOR DAMAGED SKIN

It is important to note that not all skin damage is irreversible. Rather, with intervention, certain symptoms of damage may be remedied, and almost all can be improved upon. While symptoms such as redness, dryness, uneven texture, fine lines and wrinkles, or dark spots may be treated with topical remedies (over-the-counter or prescription) or professional treatments, other more severe symptoms, such as deep wrinkles or sagging, may be best left to surgical intervention.

Despite the fact that most think of bottled products when they hear the term "skincare," the phrase actually applies to several categories, including *cosmetic surgery*, *treatment techniques*, *cosmetics*, and *skincare products*.

COSMETIC SURGERY

Surgical intervention is the only means by which one's appearance may be dramatically modified or improved. The process involves reconstruction of the cutaneous or underlying skin tissues by a board-certified plastic or cosmetic surgeon. Common examples include:

BLEPHAROPLASTY OR EYELID SURGERY

In this procedure, the excess skin and fat around the eye area is removed. It rejuvenates the adjacent skin and eliminates the tired look of aging eyes. The surgery can also correct certain functional problems like droopy eyelids and impaired vision.

BROWPLASTY OR BROW LIFT SURGERY (ALSO KNOWN AS A FOREHEAD LIFT)

A surgical approach that corrects hooded brows and the deep lines or wrinkles that appear on the forehead, browplasty imparts a more youthful and rested look and can also eradicate stern-looking or furrowed eyebrows.

CHEEK AUGMENTATION SURGERY

The aim of this procedure is to provide fullness and definition to the face. There are a wide variety of cheek implantations available, allowing the look to be customized to the patient's desired shape and size.

LIP AUGMENTATION

In this procedure, soft and pliable implants (cosmetic dermal fillers) are used to give lips a full and plump appearance.

MENTOPLASTY OR CHIN SURGERY

This procedure works to reduce, enhance, or augment the chin. By sculpting the chin and bringing it into balance with other facial structures, a more aesthetically pleasing profile may be achieved.

RHINOPLASTY OR NOSE JOB SURGERY

This procedure is conducted to change the shape of the nose. While rhinoplasty may be utilized to improve cosmetic defects, including bumps of the bridge of the nose, bulbous tips, or wide nostrils, it may also be conducted to improve nasal function, as in the case of a deviated septum.

RHYTIDECTOMY OR FACE LIFT SURGERY

Face lifts are used to address moderate to deep facial wrinkles and other natural signs of aging, including sagging facial skin. In particular, this procedure is effective on the lower two-thirds of the face.

Note: The procedures outlined above are common examples of facial plastic surgery. There are multiple additional cosmetic surgery procedures applicable to other areas of the body, including liposuction, tummy tucks, breast augmentation, and more.

IN-OFFICE TREATMENT TECHNIQUES

A number of skincare treatments are available exclusively from licensed skincare professionals or physicians, such as aestheticians, dermatologists, and plastic or cosmetic surgeons. Among the treatment techniques most often utilized to improve the condition and appearance of the skin are:

BOTOX®

A procedure that involves the injection of a prescription medicine into the frown lines between the eyes. Botox uses botulinum toxin to temporarily paralyze specific facial muscles. Within a few days of administration, Botox begins to noticeably soften wrinkles.

CHEMICAL PEELS

In this procedure a chemical solution is used to remove the damaged outer layers of facial skin, thereby improving skin texture and stimulating collagen production. Peels can be particularly beneficial in improving skin pigmentation and wrinkles and in eliminating blemishes.

DERMABRASION OR DERMAPLANING

Considered "skin refinishing" treatments, these procedures involve the removal of the skin's outermost layers via a hand-held tool. Doing so helps to remove scars and diminish wrinkles and age spots.

FILLERS

Fillers are products that are injected into the dermis or hypodermis of the skin to smooth wrinkles and restore volume loss. A wide variety of fillers are available, including those from animal sources, human sources, and synthetic materials.

LASER SKIN RESURFACING

This procedure uses pulsating beams of light to reduce wrinkles, brown spots, and enlarged pores. These improvements are due to the stimulation and tightening of collagen fibers. Laser resurfacing may also reduce hyperpigmentation.

Beyond the use of lasers for skin aesthetics, they are also used for hair removal, treating vascular lesions, tattoo removal, and more.

COSMETICS

A significant category, indeed, cosmetics have been used for more than five thousand years to temporarily hide or downplay imperfections of the skin while accentuating favorable features.

Most cosmetics are passive in nature. That is, they are functionally inactive and, therefore, won't affect the biology of the skin.

SKINCARE PRODUCTS

Skincare products are utilized to improve or maintain skin health. While some strive to achieve results similar to in-office procedures, it is important to note that most are incapable of replicating these results. Despite this, good skincare products are, indeed, capable of reducing age spots, resurfacing the skin, and stimulating collagen. For that reason, a proper home skincare regimen, utilizing effective products, is vital to extending the positive results received from in-office treatments.

Unfortunately, many companies tend to dramatize the benefits that consumers may experience from their skincare products. It is because of these marketing tactics that many consumers now expect to see miracles from overpriced products.

Among the buzz words that have sprung up in the industry in recent years is the term "cosmeceuticals." Defined as a blend of cosmetics and pharmaceuticals, cosmeceuticals feature functionally active product formulations that, therefore, impact the skin's biology in a positive manner. While cosmeceuticals are marketed as having drug-like benefits (in fact, many utilize pharmaceutical-grade ingredients), they're available over-the-counter.

Scientifically sound formulations, comprised of quality ingredients, will definitely rejuvenate the skin, to an extent, but it is essential that the limitations of these products be recognized.

Given that you now have an understanding of the composition of skin, the various factors that damage it, and some solutions to improve its appearance, let's move on to specific recommendations and guidelines for impacting overall skin health.

3

DR. A'S COMMON SENSE APPROACH TO SKINCARE

It seems as though everywhere you turn, skincare "tips" are readily being doled out. If you aren't getting them from a beauty magazine, they're coming from a friend or someone who works at the department store beauty counter. The funny thing is, so much of the instructions we receive for how to achieve beautiful skin are contradictory. For example, I've seen articles about the benefits of using a facial scrub right next to an article about avoiding abrasive cleansers. No wonder it's become so difficult to get our skin concerns under control; most people are completely confused!

Throughout the past ten-plus years I've made a point of educating my patients about the proper steps to achieving healthy skin (not *beautiful* skin, as beauty is simply a byproduct of *healthy* skin). And time after time, they're surprised at how simple it is. Like most people, they have been complicating their skincare practices by adding unnecessary steps, some of which have actually made the condition of their skin *worse*.

The skincare approach that I outline isn't groundbreaking. It doesn't require products with revolutionary new ingredients. It won't cost you a lot of money. It won't even take a lot of time. What it does do is address the needs of your skin to encourage cellular turnover, increase collagen production, eliminate and prevent dryness, even out skin tone and texture, and control blemishes and other skin imperfections. That may sound like a lot to hope for from a skincare routine. But by keeping to the basic needs of the skin, you're helping to optimize its functioning. After all, skin isn't meant to be dry, rough, or blemished. These are simply signs that it either isn't getting all that it needs or is being mistreated through the use of unnecessary products. Rather, like other organs in our body, when properly maintained, the skin can take care of itself.

The skincare routine you are about to learn is implemented daily at my skincare clinics and by my patients, at home. Together, these steps have two simple purposes: to simplify skincare while ensuring superior results. In fact, these steps form the foundation of a line of skincare products I formulated for my patients' use. Their results prove that the consistent implementation of a skincare routine designed to meet the skin's basic needs, in conjunction with healthy behaviors, can generate a marked improvement in skin health and, thus, the skin's aesthetics.

THE REGIMEN

When it comes to the products you apply to your skin, a maximum of four steps are required. In the morning, the skin should be cleansed, exfoliated, moisturized, and protected. In the evening, repeat just the cleanse, exfoliate, and moisturize steps.

STEP ONE—MORNING AND EVENING: CLEANSE

As our external defense against the outside world, the skin comes in contact with pollutants, dirt, and germs continuously throughout the day, not to mention makeup. Oil that is regularly excreted by the skin acts like a magnet, attracting and holding all that grime. Not only can this cause pores to clog, resulting in acne, the presence of bacteria can also cause infections.

Cleansing should be a part of both morning and evening skincare regimens and can be accomplished with the use of any mild soap or facial cleanser. Never use bar soap or products that contain harsh detergents, as these products can strip the skin of its natural oils.

Enough product should be used to remove buildup on the skin, which can cause bacterial growth and the decay of skin cells. It's essential that the cleanser be massaged into the skin with water long enough to ensure dirt is removed. Be cautious, however, to avoid aggressively scrubbing the skin, as this could cause irritation.

STEP TWO — MORNING AND EVENING: EXFOLIATE

As briefly discussed in chapter 2, skin undergoes a natural exfoliation process on a continual basis. As new skin cells are produced in the bottom layer of the epidermis, they migrate, flattening as they go, until they reach the outermost layer, where they are shed approximately every thirty days. This rejuvenation process is intended to heal and repair damaged skin. However, as we age, cellular turnover slows, causing the buildup of the skin's keratin layer (dead skin cells). This sets in motion a negative feedback loop whereby the skin, to protect itself from becoming too thick overall, allows its dermis to thin to accommodate the thickened keratin layer.

Among the most common side effects of unhealthy skin are those characteristics that many categorize under "sensitive skin." In reality, few individuals have truly sensitive skin. Rather, many of its symptoms, including dryness, redness, small visible blood vessels, and the like are the body's demonstration that the skin is not functioning as it should.

As you will recall, the dermis is where collagen, elastin, and other proteins are made. When it is compromised by unhealthy behaviors (improper nutrition/hydration, smoking, excessive sun exposure) or damage from aging, it begins to resemble a shantytown instead of the thriving factory it should be. In fact, if you were to look at a cross section of unhealthy skin under a microscope, you'd see thin layers due to a decrease in the amount of cells and proteins in the dermis. It would appear nearly as though the skin structure had collapsed. This weakening of the dermis layer not only causes a decrease in collagen and elastin, but it also diminishes the skin's immune response as fewer antibodies are produced. This puts the skin at risk of diseases and even skin cancer. What may be immediately noticed by individuals, however, is that their skin cannot tolerate the various products placed upon it. And, thus, it gets the label of "sensitive" rather than the "tough love" that is needed to bring it back to a healthy condition.

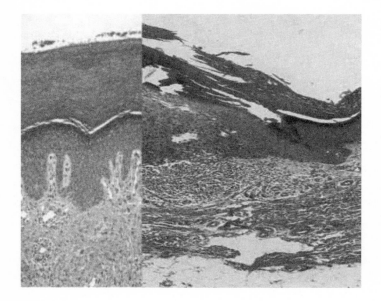

Fig. 3-1. A side-by-side comparison of normal, healthy skin, as it appears under a microscope (left) and skin that has experienced significant damage (right). Note the unorganized layers.

That tough love comes in the form of daily at-home exfoliation, which encourages skin rejuvenation. As these products dissolve the keratin layer, the skin begins producing more collagen to bring the dermis back to its proper thickness. As the health of the skin improves, it becomes noticeably more elastic, less sensitive, and, generally, more healthy looking.

Exfoliation isn't a new concept. Ancient Egyptians are credited with being the first documented civilization to exfoliate. While they relied on pumice to remove the dead layers of skin, today we have much more efficient means to encourage exfoliation. Two types of techniques may be used: mechanical or chemical. Despite the array of exfoliation products on the market today, the only way to achieve true exfoliation is via either of these methods. As mentioned in chapter 1, <u>there is absolutely no way to gently remove the thickened layers of keratin</u>. Therefore, don't waste your money and frustration purchasing products that feature "microspheres" or "granules." They fail to effectively exfoliate and, if misused, could cause inflammation, which leads to further skin damage.

MECHANICAL EXFOLIATION

Without even realizing it, most men exfoliate their faces every day through the simple act of shaving. The scraping of a blade against the skin removes dead skin layers. Observe the face of a middle-aged man who shaves regularly and you'll notice there is a disparity in the quality of the skin on the forehead and the cheek area compared to that around the jaw line. On the former you'll most likely see wrinkles and other signs of skin damage while the shaved area looks smooth and damage-free.

While mechanical exfoliation is effective, it is not very practical for at-home use. To reap the benefits, in-office procedures such as microdermabrasion, dermabrasion, or laser resurfacing are required.

CHEMICAL EXFOLIATION

The most effective way to exfoliate daily is via chemical means. Chemical exfoliation requires the use of acid to dissolve the dead keratin tissue. In the office we conduct peels to remove this layer chemically. However, it isn't realistic for patients to do an acid peel at home. Doing so would most certainly result in burns and, thus, intervention by the U.S. Food and Drug Administration (FDA) to ensure public safety. Over-the-counter acid peels do exist, but they've never been proven to offer effective exfoliation due to limitations in the amount of acid they may contain. The solution is to use an over-the-counter daily exfoliant that features an effective pH level.

A BRIEF PRIMER ON PH LEVELS

Consumers are used to seeing references to pH levels on their products, but what does "pH balanced" or "effective pH" really mean?

First, let's review how the pH scale works.

"Acidic" and "alkaline" (also called "basic") are two extremes that describe the properties of a chemical. Mixing acids and bases can cancel out or neutralize the extreme effects of the other. To measure the acidity or alkalinity of a given chemical ingredient or product, the pH scale is utilized. pH stands for "power (p) of the hydrogen (h) molecule," due to the element's role as a determinant of acidity or alkalinity. The pH scale ranges from 0 to 14 with a pH of 7 being neutral. A pH less than 7 is acidic while a pH greater than 7 is alkaline.

The pH scale is logarithmic and, as such, each whole pH value below 7 is ten times more acidic than the next higher value. For example, a pH of 5 is ten times more acidic than a pH of 6 and one hundred times (10 x 10) more acidic than a pH of 7. The same holds true for pH values above 7, each of which is ten times more alkaline than the next lower whole value. For example, a pH of 9 is ten times more alkaline than a pH of 8 and one hundred times (10 x 10) more alkaline than a pH of 7. Therefore, you can imagine that a pH of 1 is extremely acidic. Medical office peels generally have a pH around 2 or less.

The importance of a product's pH is due to its correlation to the skin's natural pH level. Human skin has a pH in the acidic range, varying from 5.5 to 6.5 depending on the individual and the area of skin tested. Acids present in the outermost layer of the epidermis determine the value of the surface pH. External factors, such as perspiration, tend to make the skin more acidic, thereby lowering the number value of the skin's pH. The higher the skin's pH number value (the less acidic it is), the greater its sensitivity reaction to acidic compounds, as characterized by burning or redness. The lower the skin's numeric pH value (the more acidic it is), the less sensitive it is to such compounds.

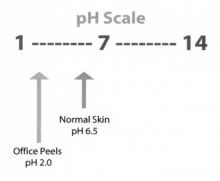

Fig. 3-2. The pH scale is used to measure acidity. A pH lower than 7 is considered acidic while a pH higher than 7 is alkaline. In-office chemical peels generally fall around a pH of 2.

Skincare products that are "pH balanced" are those formulations that have been adjusted to have, approximately, the same pH as the skin. This is beneficial in most products, including cleanser and moisturizer, as they will not disrupt the skin, causing burning or redness. However, for an exfoliation product to be effective at removing the layers of built-up keratin, an acidic pH is essential. To experience true exfoliation, an "effective pH," one that is below 3, is necessary.

The challenge with this recommendation is that many individuals will experience burning or redness if they utilize an exfoliant with a pH of 3 or below. Therefore, most skincare product formulators adjust their exfoliant's pH to be no lower than 3.5, per FDA guidelines. This is a low enough pH to provide moderate benefit. However, the best results come from an at-home exfoliant that features a pH closer to 3. This is, indeed, possible if the formulation includes a high concentration of anti-inflammatory ingredients, like aloe, which prevent burn.

ACIDS USED IN CHEMICAL EXFOLIATION

Of all the acids available, no other family of ingredients has been as beneficial in exfoliation as alpha hydroxy acids. Known simply as AHAs, these acids are naturally derived from fruits and vegetables. AHAs work by dissolving a part of the surface intercellular cement that holds keratin cells together, thus allowing them to be sloughed off.

Within the AHA family there are a variety of acids that are commonly used in skincare products and chemical peels including:

Lactic acid—derived from milk
Tartaric acid—derived from grapes and passion fruit
Malic acid—derived from apples
Glycolic acid—obtained from sugarcane or rhubarb
Citric acids—derived from citrus fruits
Retinoic acid—derived from animal sources and plants containing beta-carotene

Glycolic acid has the smallest molecules of all the

AHAs. It has been widely researched and, because of its size, penetrates between cells more readily than other acids. An added bonus—it causes the least inflammation of all the AHAs. For these reasons, it is favored in exfoliation.

A second such family is beta hydroxy acids (BHAs), which includes salicylic acid, derived from wintergreen, sweet birch, and/or willow bark. (The chemical difference between alpha and beta hydroxy acids is the location of the hydroxy acid group on the carbon chain of the acid. *Alpha* indicates that the group is on the first carbon atom, whereas *beta* demonstrates the group is on the second carbon atom.)

While AHAs and BHAs are utilized in many products, they are most effective when found in those intended to be left on the skin instead of washed off.

SELECTING AN EXFOLIATION PRODUCT

Exfoliation products each fall into one of two categories— that is, they are either effective or ineffective for the majority of the population. You would assume that manufacturers would want to create a product that falls in the former category, wouldn't you? Wrong. To be in the category whereby your product is effective for the majority of the population traditionally means your product is at risk of causing significant side effects. If a product contains a significant amount of acid, which is what is needed to garner a low pH and effective exfoliation, those who use the product are at risk of burn. To avoid this, most companies have shifted their product to the other category, whereby the product is ineffective for most users, but no one experiences negative side effects. Products that fall into this category often use either a weak acid or do contain sufficient amounts of acid in conjunction with a buffer that eats up the hydrogen ions, thus making the acid less, well, acidic. Either way, you get a higher pH level. Products such as these can be marketed as having, for example, 70% acid, a number that sounds impressive. However, they won't be very effective. This is why the pH level is so important. It's a more accurate determination of the product's strength and, therefore, effectiveness.

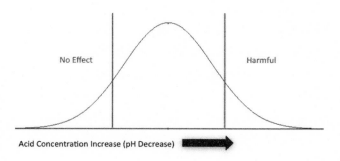

No Effect   Harmful

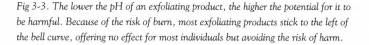

Acid Concentration Increase (pH Decrease)

Fig 3-3. The lower the pH of an exfoliating product, the higher the potential for it to be harmful. Because of the risk of burn, most exfoliating products stick to the left of the bell curve, offering no effect for most individuals but avoiding the risk of harm.

As mentioned above, the solution is to find an at-home chemical exfoliation product that features a pH closer to 3. Again, this is indeed possible and safe if the formulation includes a high concentration of anti-inflammatory ingredients, like aloe, which prevent burn.

Note that it is common for the skin to need a short period to adjust to the use of a daily exfoliant that features an effective pH. During this time you may experience dryness, flaking, slight redness, or breakouts. However, these conditions are temporary and will subside as your skin builds its tolerance to the product and becomes healthier.

FREQUENCY OF EXFOLIATION

Because the keratin layer is constantly trying to thicken, effective exfoliation is required on a daily basis, despite common recommendations that you only need to do so once per week or per month. Exfoliate that infrequently, and you'll notice the skin looks great for a short period of time after using the product. However, keratin is soon given the opportunity to thicken while the dermis thins in response. With that, dull, uneven skin tone, blemishes, and, yes, fine lines, are given the opportunity to return.

STEP THREE—MORNING AND EVENING: MOISTURIZE

As our largest organ, skin has a sizeable surface area that regularly evaporates water from inside the body in the form of sweat. Even if you aren't visibly sweating, you are. It's a basic biological function of skin. Given that skin is constantly losing moisture to the environment, it's the first part of the body to experience dehydration.

Every cell in the body is dependent upon water to maintain a healthy state. Because the skin constantly loses water by evaporation and dehydration, it becomes dry, especially in environments that are, themselves, cold and dry. It is, therefore, important to drink adequate amounts of water to prevent internal dehydration while using a moisturizer to reduce evaporation from the surface of the skin.

A common skincare myth is that water is absorbed into the skin when applied via skincare products, thus increasing moisture. This is false, as our skin cannot absorb water beyond the first few cellular layers of the epidermis. (Hopefully you've memorized the common myths from chapter 1.) Moisturizers work to *prevent* surface evaporation through the use of humectants, molecules that hold more than their weight in water and, thus, act as a barrier.

Moisturizers are essential, regardless of your skin type. Consumers with oily or acneic skin are often told that they don't need to use a moisturizer at all. What nonsense! Rather, these individuals simply need to utilize a formulation designed for their skin type.

ONE OR TWO FORMULATIONS?

Despite the common belief that you should use a separate

day and night moisturizer, this is not a necessity. Your skin does not change throughout the course of the day, requiring use of different formulations. Rather, the decision whether or not to use two separate moisturizers is a personal one.

Day moisturizers are convenient, in that they include an SPF in their formulation. This not only saves a step in the morning skincare routine, it also ensures your skin is protected. Night moisturizers are not only absent an SPF, they are also often formulated with additional humectants and masking agents to make them more moisturizing (and heavier) than their daytime counterparts.

A WORD OF CAUTION WHEN SELECTING A MOISTURIZER

Moisturizers tend to be the skincare product in which consumers most appreciate a pleasing smell and product texture. Because of this, skincare brands often load their products with fragrances and other ingredients to appeal to consumers' senses. Therefore, I caution you against selecting a moisturizer, or any skincare product for that matter, by simply testing the product on your hand or choosing it based on smell. It's far too easy to be swayed by a product's aesthetics. Remember, it's a product's formulation that matters.

STEP FOUR—MORNING: PROTECT

Thankfully, consumers today are well aware of the dangers that ultraviolet light present to the skin. Not only does UV light pose a potential cancer threat, it is also one of the main causes of skin damage.

As just mentioned, most of today's moisturizers for daily use include SPF in their formulations. Therefore, the "protect" step is often integrated within that of "moisturize." This is beneficial since the risks from sun exposure are consistent year-round. Sunscreen should be applied every single day, regardless of your skin tone.

But relying on the sunscreen in your facial moisturizer isn't enough to ensure adequate protection for your skin. When outdoors for extended periods of time, protective clothing and the application of a sunscreen with an SPF of at least 15 to exposed areas of skin should be routine. (Numerous studies have demonstrated that sunscreens with an SPF greater than 30 offer only a minimal increase in protection. SPF 30 protects you from 95 to 96% of UV rays. Between SPF 30 and SPF 60, for example, there is only a .1% increase in protection.)

ADDED BENEFITS OF THE REGIMEN

The four-step regimen is essential in that it meets the skin's primary needs of keeping pores clear, promoting efficient cellular turnover and rejuvenation, preventing the excessive loss of moisture, and staying protected from UV light. But consistently implementing the regimen has an added benefit: It helps the skin counter inflammation and oxidation, two factors that significantly contribute to skin damage.

INFLAMMATION

The body's response to harmful stimuli—including trauma, irritation, harmful pollutants, disease, or infection—inflammation is an immune response intended to protect and heal. We are all familiar with the symptoms associated with the onset of inflammation, including redness, warmth, swelling, and pain, all of which occur due to the increase in blood flow to the area and the release of chemicals intended to fight off offending events. However, chronic inflammation is believed to be the root cause of many diseases, including heart disease, cancer, and Alzheimer's. In fact, it has been implicated as one of, if not the biggest, causes of aging.[3] It should therefore come as no surprise that inflammation promotes signs of aging in the skin. This is because inflammation inflicts collateral damage as it defends the body.

If any of the basic needs of the skin are not met, the onset of inflammation is encouraged. Skin isn't properly cleaned? The presence of bacteria causes inflammation. Skin isn't properly exfoliated? The dermis layer thins and skin is more easily damaged, leading to inflammation. Skin isn't properly moisturized? Inflammation begins in an attempt to heal dry skin. Skin isn't properly protected? You increase your risk of sunburn, which causes inflammation.

Many skincare products for use within the four steps are formulated with ingredients to offset inflammation. Key ingredients to look for include aloe vera, one of the most potent anti-inflammatories available; bisbolol; green tea extract; and arnica.

OXIDATION

While oxygen is essential to the human body in that it enables our cells to harness energy from the food we eat, it also has the potential to cause harm. When molecules within cells encounter oxygen from internal factors, like breathing and metabolism, as well as those external, most notably excessive sun exposure, pollution, cigarette smoke, and more, a reaction occurs and a free radical is produced. This process is called oxidation.

Free radicals, which can also be formed during the natural aging process, are unstable atoms or molecules, characterized by at least one unpaired electron. Thus, the free radical steals electrons from nearby molecules within the cell, turning them, too, into free radicals. It's a chain reaction that causes increasing damage to the cells of the body. As this free radical cascade continues, it can lead to disease. For example, free radicals are a suggested cause of heart disease, Parkinson's disease, and even cancer. And, like inflammation, they're also believed to be a leading cause of aging.[4] In skin, free radicals lead to the breakdown of collagen and elastin, resulting in the development of fine lines and wrinkles.

Luckily, antioxidants act like soldiers for our cells. They provide electrons to free radicals, thereby disabling them and preventing cell damage. This, in turn, prevents damage to skin tissue. There are thousands of known antioxidants, which fall into several antioxidant categories, including carotenoids, flavonoids, and polyphenols.

In 2009, a team of fellow researchers and I implemented a study to determine if antioxidants found in moisturizers can, indeed, increase the antioxidant levels within the skin.[5] That study proved that antioxidant formulations are, indeed, beneficial as long as they can be absorbed. In the next chapter, we'll review the building blocks of skincare formulations so you can determine those products that are more readily absorbed by the skin.

Because inclusion of antioxidants in skincare formulations has become a hot topic today, it's easy to find products for use within the four steps that utilize them. Key ingredients to look for include vitamin C (L-ascorbic acid), vitamin E, coenzyme Q10, and alpha lipoic acid.

GARNERING HEALTHY SKIN FROM THE INSIDE

While use of skincare products that meet the skin's basic needs are essential, this is just half of the formula to achieve healthy skin. As you will recall from chapter 2, skin is a water-resistant, semi-impermeable barrier. Therefore, skincare products applied topically don't fully improve the skin, especially if the products are water-based. Delivering vitamins, minerals, fats, and proteins to the skin through nutrition is essential. In fact, if you cannot ensure a healthy diet, the best skincare products in the world won't benefit you whatsoever. Skin health *begins* from the inside.

While the intention of this book is not to outline a diet plan to ensure healthy skin, there are a number of nutrients that are especially important in this quest. Among them:

Protein, which encourages the production of collagen and aids in cellular repair.

Essential fatty acids, which nourish the skin, including Omega-3 fats to help reduce inflammation and mono-unsaturated fats to help reduce oxidative damage.

Antioxidants to help prevent damage to skin tissue.

It's advantageous to fill the bulk of your diet with fruits and vegetables, legumes, fish, healthy oils (e.g. olive oil), and whole grains while significantly limiting the consumption of refined sugar and carbohydrates. In fact, several studies have shown that consumption of meat, dairy, fats, and carbohydrates may actually promote skin wrinkling.[6; 7]

The use of some supplements may be beneficial in ensuring your skin receives the proper level of nutrients. While there are many formulations designed specifically for healthier skin, I believe there is no need for anything more than a daily vitamin.

And, of course, there's the issue of hydration. As stated earlier, it is necessary to drink adequate amounts of water to prevent internal dehydration. The cells of the body, skin cells included, require moisture to function properly.

Even if you faithfully follow the four-step regimen, eat a healthy diet, and ensure proper hydration, it's impossible to avoid all causes of skin damage. The natural process of aging, alone, will cause our skin to wrinkle. However, implementation of the principles outlined here will significantly improve the health of your skin and minimize environmental damage factors.

Remember—skin must be treated as the vital organ that it is. And the very best approach is one of simplicity and common sense.

4

SIMPLIFIED DECODING OF THE BOTTLE

Next to fragrances, skincare products are among the most beautifully packaged items in a department store. Once you are lured by the packaging design, it only takes a dab of the product to be sold by the attractive scent or the silky texture. Skincare products are often more about the aesthetics of the product than the aesthetics of your skin.

Because of this, it's necessary for customers to have the ability to protect themselves from buying products that don't work or could even cause adverse effects and, instead, be equipped with the knowledge to select those that will improve the condition of their skin. The FDA currently does not approve cosmetics, the category in which skincare products are placed, before they go to market as they do drugs. They also don't regulate most of the ingredients used in skincare formulations. Simply put, no one is watching out for you all that closely.

Beyond ensuring you select a quality product, understanding the basics of skincare formulations allows you to:

> Avoid products that contain known irritants or allergens.
> Purchase products that contain ingredients proven beneficial in skincare applications.
> Eliminate the clutter in your medicine cabinet by helping you identify useless products.

To understand formulations you don't need to pull out your old chemistry textbooks. Rather, you must simply know the role of each category that comprises skincare products, what to look for within the categories, and ingredients that are best avoided. Also, once you know your particular skin type, you can look for ingredients that are proven to improve your specific skin concerns.

THE BUILDING BLOCKS OF SKINCARE PRODUCTS

Skincare products, to be safe and effective, must be formulated through a delicate balance of chemicals and components, each added at the proper time and in the appropriate concentration and quality.

Most skincare products are *passive* in character. This means that they do nothing to physically stimulate skin functioning—an important point, indeed, if your goal is to have your skincare product actually improve your skin. Marketing often leads one to believe that products are capable of bringing about significant improvements to the skin after just a few days of use. In reality, however, improvement is only possible if the product houses an appropriate amount of *active* agents.

ACTIVE SKINCARE AGENTS

Active skincare agents enhance cellular repair by stimulating and improving naturally occurring skin functions. Among the many abilities of active ingredients, they may reflect, scatter, or block UV light, as in sunscreens; exfoliate, thus stimulating the production of collagen; lighten skin pigmentation; and prevent cellular damage, as in antioxidant formulations.

The most commonly utilized active skincare agents include:

> › Alpha hydroxy acids, including glycolic acid, lactic acid, and citric acid
> › Amino acids
> › Anti-inflammatories, including aloe vera and bisabolol

> Antioxidants, including L-ascorbic acid, alpha lipoic acid, tocopherol, and copper peptide
> Beta hydroxy acids, including salicylic acid
> Lightening agents, like hydroquinone and kojic acid
> Lipids, including ceramides
> Retinoids (forms of vitamin A), including retinol and tretinoin
> Vitamins and vitamin-like substances, including niacinamide and ubiquinone, commonly known as coenzyme Q10

PASSIVE SKINCARE AGENTS

My emphasis on the vital role of active agents should not downplay the important role that passive agents play in skincare.

Passive agents comprise the majority of the ingredients in a skincare product and are necessary for ensuring the active ingredients get to the site of skin healing. For example, at home you wouldn't be able to simply apply glycolic acid to your skin to promote exfoliation. While glycolic acid is applied directly to skin as part of professional chemical peels, it would most certainly burn your skin if used outside the spa or medical office. For at-home exfoliation, two methods are used to ensure a product's safety: 1) glycolic acid is blended with passive ingredients to neutralize the acid and 2) a strong anti-inflammatory agent is utilized. Supplementary ingredients also ensure the product maintains its composition, has a consistency that is easily applied, and penetrates skin.

Whether active or passive in nature, the ingredient categories that comprise skincare products may include:

BASE: THE MAIN INGREDIENT

The main ingredient of any skincare product, the *base,* is tasked with carrying the other ingredients used in the formulation to the site of skin healing and rejuvenation (it acts as the "delivery vehicle" for the formulation). Of course, this means the base ingredient needs to be capable of penetrating skin.

Most skincare products use a base of water. After all, it's abundant and inexpensive, making it an excellent base—from a manufacturer's perspective. However, the skin cannot absorb water. (If it did, we wouldn't be able to swim!) While a small amount does get absorbed into the keratin layer—the cause of wrinkly skin after a bath—it does not reach the layers where skin healing and rejuvenation occur. Therefore, the active ingredients in the formulation aren't able to provide their intended benefit. In fact, the presence of water only dilutes the other ingredients.

Instead, it's beneficial to look for a product that features a therapeutic base capable of penetrating deep into the skin, thereby carrying other active ingredients with it. One such base is aloe vera. An active ingredient, aloe has potent anti-inflammatory abilities and, therefore, helps eliminate symptoms of inflammation-based skin conditions, including acne, dermatitis, and rosacea. What's more, aloe is able to penetrate the skin. When administered in the appropriate concentrations of the highest quality, the benefits of an aloe-based formulation are apparent nearly immediately.

AESTHETIC ADDITIVES

Among the ingredients added to a skincare formulation to improve its aesthetics are colorings and fragrances. These additives may be utilized to mask the natural scent or color of the formulation's ingredients (which may be unappealing, albeit effective). Most often, however, fragrances and colorings are used to improve a product's psychological appeal.

Fragrances are one of the leading causes of allergies from skincare products. In fact, nearly six percent of the human population is allergic to fragrances.

ANTIOXIDANTS

An overview of antioxidants was outlined in chapter 3. As discussed, they protect our cells from free radical damage. Because our body produces fewer antioxidants as we age, their presence in anti-aging formulations is particularly beneficial.

Among the antioxidants to look for in skincare products are L-ascorbic acid, coenzyme Q10, alpha lipoic acid, and vitamin E.

BIOLOGICAL ADDITIVES

Biological additives are derived from a biological source and mainly utilized to improve the aesthetics of a product, including its look, feel, and smell. While they are generally not active ingredients, we're learning more about biological additives and discovering that some may have active properties. Research into the potential of biological additives is currently an exciting topic in the skincare products industry.

Examples of biological additives include extracts of grains, flowers, and fruits, as well as collagen and elastin.

SUNBLOCKS

Sunblocks ensure mechanical protection from the sun's ultraviolet rays by covering the skin. Thus, they provide complete protection.

Blocks include zinc oxide and titanium dioxide.

EMOLLIENTS

Emollients are added to skincare formulations to "lock in" natural moisture and protect the skin by placing a protective barrier on its surface. (A more appropriate term for them is "moisturizer.") Aesthetically, emollients leave the surface of the skin feeling temporarily softer and smoother. Common emollients used in skincare formulations include cetyl alcohol, glycerin, panthenol, and dimethicone.

EMULSIFYING AGENTS

Emulsifiers help to blend the water- and oil-soluble components of a formulation. The most commonly used emulsifying agents are glycereth 20, carbomer, isopropyl palmitate, and polysorbate.

EXFOLIANTS

Exfoliants are active chemicals that dissolve away keratin, the built-up layers of dead skin and debris. Although exfoliants promote normal skin growth, they are seldom found to have a positive impact in direct healing or wound repair. Potent exfoliants include glycolic acid and salicylic acid.

HUMECTANTS

Humectants are chemical substances that can absorb water. As such, humectants are utilized in skincare products to aid in the prevention of moisture loss from the surface of the skin. When selecting a moisturizer, it is essential that its formulation contain humectants to be effective.

The most commonly used humectants include propylene glycol, lanolin, sorbitol, urea, glycerin, and hyaluronic acid.

PRESERVATIVES

Preservatives are added to formulations to prevent contamination by bacteria. Without them, consumers would be at significant risk when using products that are applied to the skin.

Common preservatives used in skincare formulations include parabens (such as methylparaben, polyparaben, and butylparaben), imidazolydyl urea, and phenoxyethanol.

SUNSCREENS

Sunscreens selectively absorb ultraviolet light. They are semi-active, in that the chemicals of the screen may interact with the cells and actively prevent ultraviolet damage to them. The measurement by which sunscreens prevent ultraviolet damage is referred to as the Sun Protection Factor (SPF). SPF 15 offers protection from 92% of damaging UV rays. Contrary to popular belief, higher numbered SPFs only increase protection minimally. No screen offers complete protection.

Examples of sunscreens include methoxycinnamate and oxybenzone. When selecting a sunscreen product, be sure to look for one that offers broad-spectrum protection, as these will protect from both UVA and UVB rays.

SOLVENTS

Solvents are used to help a skincare product reach its proper consistency. They may dissolve or suspend another ingredient without changing the chemical makeup of either property.

Common solvents in skincare products include propylene glycol, glycerin, various oils (e.g. soybean oil), and, most commonly, water.

SURFACTANTS

Surfactants are used to dissolve dirt and oil present on the skin or to act as a lubricant in a skincare product. They work by reducing the surface tension of a liquid.

In skincare products, the most commonly utilized surfactants include sodium laureth sulfate, sodium stearate, and sodium palmitate.

INGREDIENT GRADES

It is possible for skincare formulations to feature the same collection of ingredients in similar concentrations but still offer different results. This is because of differences in ingredient grades. All ingredients fall into one of five grades. In descending order, these are pharmaceutical, food, cosmetic, reagent, and technical. In skincare products cosmetic-grade is most commonly utilized. In fact, it is this grade that is commonly utilized in skincare products found at drug and department stores. While there is certainly nothing wrong with cosmetic grade ingredients, they are less refined than higher grade ingredients and, thereby, contain impurities.

(The FDA allows up to 30% impurities in cosmetic-grade ingredients.) Many skincare products, however, utilize ingredients of the highest quality—pharmaceutical grade, which are required to be 99.9% pure.

Often, formulations that utilize pharmaceutical-grade ingredients will highlight this in the ingredient list. If you aren't sure, however, it's beneficial to call the company's customer service number to find out what grades they utilize.

TRANSLATING INGREDIENT LISTS

Despite the fact that the FDA does not approve skincare products, they provide some protection for consumers via the Fair Packaging and Labeling Act. This law requires manufacturers to follow specific criteria when developing product labels, including listing product ingredients in the order of concentration. Additionally, all ingredients must be listed by their INCI name, that is, the International Nomenclature of Cosmetic Ingredients. The INCI outlines the appropriate scientific term for each ingredient. For example, it takes a simple ingredient like shea butter and requires it be listed as Butyrospermum Parkii (Shea Butter). While this may seem to make labels more difficult to read, it ensures that labels read consistently across languages and cultures.

So, then, what are the steps to reading an ingredient label and, ultimately, selecting a skincare product?

STEP 1:

Look at the ingredient list. Is the first item (the base ingredient) water, or is it a therapeutic healing agent, such as aloe vera? Higher consideration should be given to the latter.

STEP 2:

Do you see any active ingredients listed in the ingredient list? Also, is there more than one active ingredient included in the formulation? The higher on the list the active ingredient falls, the more concentrated it is in the formulation. Many active ingredients work well in small concentrations, while others, like aloe, must be included in high concentrations to be effective. It's, therefore, important to research active ingredients in a formulation to understand how they're best utilized while determining the potential for side effects. Some active ingredients may be irritating in higher concentrations until the skin has adapted to their presence.

STEP 3:

Do you see any harsh chemicals listed, such as acetone, camphor, fennel, menthol, rubbing alcohol, or phenol? Ingredients such as these are considered irritants. Exposure to irritants may cause a variety of conditions that are difficult to treat, including redness, dry patches, breakouts, rashes, flakiness, and sensitivity.

Today there are countless products claiming to improve the condition of our skin while containing irritating ingredients. The use of these products may cause the skin to swell temporarily, ultimately leading to wrinkles and premature aging. Repeated use can even suppress the skin's immune and healing response by breaking down intercellular chambers. Therefore, these products don't provide benefits. Instead, they do damage.

STEP 4:

Does the product contain pharmaceutical-grade ingredients? As mentioned, if they do it will usually be highlighted on the packaging.

HOT BUTTON INGREDIENTS

Of course, unless you're a chemist by trade, product ingredient lists can be overwhelming. For that reason, I advise you to research the individual ingredients in product formulations. And what better tool to do that than the Internet? However, relying on the web to learn more about ingredients can be both beneficial and detrimental. It seems there are both "pro" and "con" camps for nearly every skincare ingredient. Often, these campaigns are plagued by misinformation. This is why decisions about skincare formulations must be based on the findings of clinical studies instead of Internet rumors.

Examples of ingredients that have come under scrutiny include:

SODIUM LAURETH SULFATE

A surfactant (detergent) used in cleansers, sodium laureth sulfate came under scrutiny in the late 90s when an Internet rumor began circulating about the "carcinogenic" nature of this ingredient. Despite the inaccuracy of the rumor, sodium laureth sulfate was soon villainized.

The truth is, those with particularly sensitive skin should avoid sodium laureth sulfate, as it can be irritating. But for the majority of the population, the ingredient poses negligible risk.

MINERAL OIL

When mineral oil first began being used in moisturizers, it proved to be an excellent humectant. This led to the unfortunate assumption that if a little mineral oil provides beneficial results, using a lot in a formulation will make it even better. However, when used in high concentrations, mineral oil can plug pores, leading to acne and diminished skin health. Improper use of mineral oil led to the unfortunate widespread belief that *any* use of the ingredient in a skincare formulation is bad.

To be beneficial in a skincare formulation, mineral oil must be used in limited concentration and must be of cosmetic grade or higher (pharmaceutical grade is best). The lesser the grade, the more impurities it may have. However, considering that the FDA regulates the purity level of mineral oil, there's a slim chance of finding a poor grade in your skincare product.

A second rumor about mineral oil is that it causes cancer. This report is completely baseless, as no scientific study has ever indicated a link between mineral oil and cancer.

ALCOHOL

Alcohol is the ingredient that I absolutely recommend you avoid using in skincare products. It is often found in "toners" to help remove dirt and give the skin a refreshed feeling. However, alcohol is an irritant and dries the skin. This causes inflammation and increases the risk of skin damage.

It is important to note that there are some beneficial skincare ingredients that are related to alcohol, including glycols, which act as emollients. The fats and oils found in glycols moisturize the skin. When these fatty acids are removed, the result is alcohol.

Try to avoid products that list alcohol in forms like ethyl alcohol and isopropyl alcohol, as well as ethanol and methanol.

UREA

Urea is a preservative commonly used in skincare products. The reasons propagated for not using it are twofold. There are those who say it is a waste byproduct of the body, making it unappealing for use in skincare products. And then there's the group who says urea releases formaldehyde and is, therefore, a carcinogen. Here's the real deal:

It's true that urea is a waste produced when the body metabolizes protein. However, the urea used in skincare products is not the same chemical and comes from a synthetic process. Therefore, you can rest assured you aren't applying waste products to your face.

Regarding the risk of cancer from using products with urea, this is a completely unfounded assertion. In fact, in 1990, the FDA asked its Cosmetic Ingredient Review (CIR) Expert Panel to review the science on urea. That investigation led to a report stating that urea is, indeed, safe for use in cosmetics in concentrations up to 0.5 percent. In 2006, the CIR again investigated urea, using current science. That investigation led to a report that confirmed the findings from 1990 and again declared urea safe for use in cosmetics. (You can find an overview of ingredients the CIR has investigated at www.cir-safety.org.)

PARABENS

Of all the controversial skincare ingredients, it's the topic of parabens that I'm most passionate about. And, for that reason, I want to elaborate on it a bit more than some of the other ingredients.

As a plastic surgeon who has had countless breast cancer survivors as patients, I'm particularly sensitive to ingredients that are considered carcinogenic—especially those that may be linked to breast cancer, specifically. Therefore, in 2004, when the Internet began swirling with claims that parabens cause cancer, I immediately dove into the research to get the full story. After all, parabens are among the most utilized preservatives in the skincare industry and have been used safely and effectively for more than eighty years. If they were suddenly found dangerous, countless skincare products would be affected.

Here's the background:

In 2004, a researcher in the United Kingdom named Phillipa Darbre published a study in the Journal of Applied Toxicology that found paraben-like substances in breast cancer tissue.[8] Given the sensitivity in our society to breast cancer, it didn't take long for parabens to be put at the top of every list of "bad skincare products." Additionally, skincare product manufacturers almost immediately began changing their formulations to utilize newer preservatives.

What the Darbre study did not do is show causation of breast cancer by parabens. It also failed to show them to be harmful in any way. In fact, the study left many questions unanswered. For example, it did not look at possible paraben levels in normal tissue, an essential step if any valid conclusion was to be made.

Since the Darbre study, follow-up investigations, including a 2008 comprehensive review by the Cosmetic Ingredient Review (CIR), have confirmed parabens' safety. With that, the FDA, the National Cancer Institute, and the American Cancer Society, among others, released statements denying proof of a linkage between parabens and breast cancer. Today, parabens remain officially approved for use in cosmetics by the U.S. FDA, the European Commission, the Japanese Ministry of Health, Labour and Welfare, and many more regulatory bodies. Despite this, the fear campaign surrounding parabens continues, spurred on by various special interest groups and even manufacturers who have turned to paraben-free preservatives.

So what's wrong with using an alternative preservative in skincare products? Perhaps nothing. However, we can't be sure because most other preservatives are relatively new and lack the long track record of success that accompanies parabens.

What is most alarming is that the paraben controversy, and others like it, have led some manufacturers to condemn preservatives altogether and, with that, they've begun marketing "preservative-free" formulations. Nearly every skincare product on the market today contains some amount of water. And with the use of water comes risk, for it creates a habitat in which bacteria, fungi, molds, and other microorganisms are encouraged to grow and thrive. Thus, there can be no such thing as a preservative-free skincare product unless it is to have no shelf life or is exclusively oil-based or water-free.

Rather, there are many ways to mask the presence of man-made preservatives. And it is of this issue that I've found few to be aware. In fact, natural/organic preservative distributors will even admit that a truly natural broad spectrum preservative is not currently available.

While there are some "natural" substances that offer antibacterial benefits at high concentrations, such as certain essential oils, they are very narrow in their spectrum of protection against bacteria. The challenge is that there is no way to add these preservatives in high enough concentrations without causing severe reactions. And conversely, adding an amount that will avoid irritation doesn't offer protection from microorganisms.

Of the many natural preservatives utilized in skincare products today, a good number have failed challenge testing by third-party groups such as the Cosmetic Toiletry Fragrance Association (CTFA) or United States Pharmacopeia (USP). Despite this, manufacturers continue to use the ingredients and back them by claiming they passed the company's own internal testing requirements. Additionally, some "preservative-free" skincare products utilize a loophole to hide the presence of preservatives. The FDA does not require manufacturers to disclose the actual ingredients that comprise "fragrance" or "parfum." Therefore, companies are able to include preservatives in their products but mask their presence with the "fragrance" umbrella. This is also sometimes done with the ingredient terms "base" or "blend."

The fact is, preservatives that are found freely in nature may be more irritating since they do not conform to the rules that are applied to the ingredients used in product formulations. Skincare products require stability and shelf life, and, unfortunately, natural preservatives aren't very adapting to those requirements. The simple fact is that man-made formulations have fewer by-products and are, thus, safer than natural biologically active ingredients.

Ensuring skincare formulations do more than simply smell or feel nice does require some work on your part. However, it's a worthy effort, indeed. The time you invest will save you money and frustration. More important, however, it will bring a sense of satisfaction when your effort leads you to a product that provides an undeniable improvement in the condition of your skin.

5

ALOE: THE POWERHOUSE INGREDIENT

Of all the ingredients used in skincare formulations, there is one that I hold paramount: aloe. That often comes as a surprise to my patients. After all, like you, they're used to seeing aloe featured in thousands of products—from lotions and shaving cream to dish soap and even toilet paper—that they take its abilities for granted. But don't underestimate this powerhouse ingredient. When used properly in skincare formulations, aloe can bring a marked improvement to skin.

As mentioned in an earlier chapter, I had the advantage of receiving my surgical training under some of the world's leading aloe researchers, including Dr. Martin Robson, who pioneered much of the research into the plant's healing abilities. It is because of his work that I today utilize high-grade aloe in my practice. While I regularly apply pure aloe to surgical flaps to expedite healing, it is also used by my staff, who apply aloe-based products to patient skin pre- and post-non-surgical procedures, such as chemical peels, microdermabrasion, and laser procedures. Regardless of the skincare scenario, aloe provides a benefit.

ALOE HISTORY

Aloe has been used medicinally for countless centuries by numerous world civilizations. In fact, records of its restorative powers can be found on Sumerian clay tablets dating back to 2100 BC. Even Cleopatra is said to have regularly used aloe, regarding it as her "beauty secret." The documented ancient uses for aloe included treatment of sinus pain, burns, wounds, and infections, to name a few.

Prior to embarking on his quest for world domination, Alexander the Great sought counsel by famed Greek physician and philosopher Aristotle, who instructed him to be sure to conquer the Isle of Socotra (modern day Yemen) to collect what he called "the potted physician"—aloe plants that could be used to help heal the wounds of his troops. And, indeed, aloe is beneficial even today on the battlefield. Researchers from the University of Pittsburgh published a study in 2004 that showed juice of the aloe plant could keep war casualties or other trauma victims alive until they could receive a blood transfusion.[9]

Scientific research into the healing abilities of aloe is relatively new, however. The first study occurred in 1935 when Collins and Collins discovered it to be beneficial in the treatment of radiation dermatitis (radio-dermatitis), a disease caused by exposure to radiation. Since then, countless studies have proven aloe's clinical effectiveness in treating a wide range of conditions, including superficial skin abrasions, frostbite, psoriasis, burns, periodontal disease, peptic ulcers, herpes, and even asthma. In fact, I've personally had the privilege of leading several research studies that demonstrated aloe's abilities in wound healing[10] and in the treatment of specific diabetic conditions.[11] Each day, new discoveries surrounding aloe's healing abilities occur. In fact, it is one of the few natural substances scientifically proven to heal the body.

THE ROLE OF ALOE IN SKINCARE

Aloe's healing elements are found in the plant's yellow-green gel, which oozes from its fleshy stalks. Here, more than two hundred active components can be found, including vitamins, minerals, amino acids, enzymes, polysaccharides, fatty acids, and more. While science is still uncovering the healing potential of aloe, its key abilities, as they relate to skincare, include:

ALOE PENETRATES TISSUE.

Unlike water, aloe can be absorbed by the skin. In fact, it is absorbed deep into its layers. This is due to the presence of lignin, a substance similar to cellulose. Lignin allows the active components of the plant to be delivered to the site of healing. Additionally, it ensures that other active ingredients present in aloe-based skincare formulations are delivered within the skin's layers.

ALOE ACTS AS AN ANESTHETIC.

Aloe has a high magnesium content and contains aspirin-like compounds. Therefore, it is commonly used to alleviate the pain of burns and wounds, including countless skin ailments. Of course, it is this characteristic that most recognize in aloe. Consumers most popularly use it for the treatment of sunburn.

ALOE HAS ANTIMICROBIAL PROPERTIES.

Among the antimicrobial compounds found in aloe are saponin, which acts as an antiseptic, and barbaloin, an effective antimicrobial. Given that bacteria are a main cause of acne, aloe's antimicrobial properties are beneficial in treatment of the condition.

ALOE IS AN ANTI-INFLAMMATORY.

Aloe contains numerous components that provide it with anti-inflammatory abilities, including salicylic acid (a beta hydroxy acid), sterols, and enzymes. Nearly all skin conditions, including acne and the telltale signs of aging, stem from inflammation, making aloe an ideal remedy.

ALOE IS PROVEN TO HEAL WOUNDS.

Scientific research has shown that several components in aloe are responsible for the substance's excellent ability to regenerate cells. These include gibberellin, a growth hormone-like substance that increases protein synthesis, and lectin, a protein that increases collagen activity. Thus, aloe may be utilized to heal conditions, such as acne or eczema, while improving the overall health and structure of the skin.

ALOE IS MOISTURIZING.

Not only does aloe soothe the skin, but it also has moisturizing capabilities, due to the polysaccharide content within the plant.

OPTIMIZING THE BENEFITS OF ALOE IN SKINCARE

While aloe is readily available in nearly every type of skincare product—from cleansers and serums to moisturizers and sunscreens—few, if any of these products deliver the benefits outlined above. Why? Because most products utilize aloe of improper quality and concentration. To experience the healing benefits of aloe, skincare formulations must follow a set of rules:

IT'S A MATTER OF CONCENTRATION.

Aloe must be used in high concentrations to ensure its benefits will be realized. As stated in an earlier chapter, in order to achieve this, aloe should be used as the product's base ingredient. As such, it will be the first ingredient listed on the back of the product. Most often, it's water that you'll find listed in this primary role.

A base of water dilutes the active ingredients in a product, which makes any aloe it does contain virtually worthless. Additionally, water-based products are essentially non-therapeutic. To make them therapeutic, medicines must be added to the product formula, which often puts consumers at risk of adverse side effects. Conversely, aloe-based products are therapeutic by their very nature.

Given aloe's ability to penetrate deep into the skin's layers (unlike water, which cannot be absorbed), it is an excellent carrier for other effective ingredients. Therefore, beyond the need to have a high concentration in order to experience its benefits, a base of aloe offers additional advantages.

BEYOND QUANTITY, THERE'S QUALITY.

Like other cosmetic ingredients, aloe is available in a range of grades, as outlined in chapter 4. In addition to the numerous beneficial components present in aloe, the plant also contains active ingredients considered impurities because of their capacity to cause contact irritation or allergic reactions in some individuals. Given that cosmetic-grade ingredients can have up to 30% impurities, per the FDA, cosmetic-grade aloe may actually be detrimental to some skin types. For this reason, it is necessary to select a product that utilizes pharmaceutical-grade aloe, which is 99.9% pure.

Beyond the grade of aloe, there are also two main types that are used in skincare products. These include "whole leaf" and "inner fillet."

Whole leaf aloe is made by grinding both the interior and outer rind of the aloe leaf, while inner fillet aloe is made by removing the outer rind of the leaf and harvesting only the interior of the stalk. Aloe gel made from whole leaf is less expensive but is subjected to more processing. Thus, it contains more undesirable materials. While whole leaf aloe is often used, nearly all research conducted on aloe's benefits was done using inner fillet. Therefore, when looking to garner benefits from an aloe-based product, it is advantageous to use one that features inner fillet.

QUALITY STARTS AT THE FARM.

Aloe's active ingredients begin to break down and lose their effectiveness immediately after harvesting, a situation that is only compounded by inferior processing. When aloe leaves are crushed, an enzyme is activated that begins to kill off the mannose molecules in aloe, essential sugars that are key to aloe's healing abilities. In time, this enzyme will digest all of aloe's beneficial polysaccharides as a termite digests wood.

To avoid this decomposition of benefits, aloe must be processed quickly within four to six hours of harvesting. This ensures the harvested aloe retains its "bioactivity." In other words, it maintains its therapeutic healing properties and will work synergistically with the body's own healing mechanisms. Additionally, effective processing requires that aloe's molecular structure be stabilized, standardized, freeze-dried, and ground to a powder or created into a gel—all within that short window of opportunity.

So how can you ensure these guidelines have been properly followed in the aloe contained in your skincare product line? The International Aloe Science Council (IASC), a non-profit trade organization dedicated to providing the world with the highest quality of aloe, is the governing body that certifies high-quality aloe. By looking for the IASC seal (or purchasing products that utilize IASC-certified

aloe) you can rest assured that the aloe contained in a product meets only the most stringent quality standards.

FRESH ALOE VS.
PHARMACEUTICAL GRADE

Now, given all that you've learned about the benefits of aloe,
you may be tempted to simply keep a plant on your counter
for direct application to the skin. However, it's necessary to
note that the exceptional results noted in clinical research
cannot be replicated through the use of fresh aloe. House-
hold aloe is a different species than the Aloe barbadensis
Miller that is used in skincare and medical applications.
And don't forget that unprocessed aloe contains irritating
substances that could do more harm than good.

Despite this, I've heard countless personal accounts of
individuals using an aloe plant on small wounds and burns,
to much success. But for optimal skincare, skip the stalk,
and, instead, look for products that use premium aloe.

While today the list of skincare lines that feature aloe-
based products is relatively small, recent research has
opened the eyes of many formulators to the benefits of using
it. For that reason, I expect in coming years we'll see a significant increase in the number of brands that transition
from water-based to aloe-based products. This is, indeed,
beneficial to the skincare category, overall. However, it's

essential that when shopping for aloe-based skincare products, you ensure they follow the "rules" outlined above. Products that utilize aloe improperly won't provide the same benefits and, thus, will only be a waste of your money.

6

COMMON SKIN CONCERNS

You can tell a lot about a person by simply looking at their face. I don't mean their expressions, but rather, their skin. Bad habits like poor nutrition, improper skincare, excessive tanning, or regular smoking all leave calling cards. While certain habits can cause long-term concerns, such as premature aging or, worse, cancer, most result in nagging issues that can be improved by simply ceasing the behavior or improving it.

Of course, a large portion of skin conditions, concerns, and damage are also caused by factors of which we have no control, like aging, medical conditions, and heredity. Yet, even in these cases, there are often solutions that can minimize the symptoms, if not eliminate them. That's where this chapter comes in. In addition to outlining the various causes of common skin concerns, I present an overview of the various treatment options available.

First, a word about my approach to these skincare issues. Read five different skincare books and you'll often find five different approaches for treating common skin concerns. This is because rarely is there just one way to treat the skin. Various protocols can get you to the same end result of improved skin appearance. However, my philosophy is to utilize proven tactics of addressing the issue to bring about a noticeable improvement in appearance and, most importantly, a measurable impact on the skin's health. After all, this method offers the best defense against symptoms reoccurring.

My approach is one of minimal invasiveness. Of course, many skin concerns can be immediately alleviated through plastic surgery or cosmetic procedures. However, I look at these options as those to consider when all others fail to improve the situation. Therefore, within the pages of this chapter, I outline both at-home and over-the-counter solutions for the most common skin challenges and conditions, as well as the appropriate professional procedures that may address them. These suggested treatments are based on sound scientific research and successful results that have been garnered in my practice.

DRYNESS

Skin dryness may be caused by a variety of scenarios. In fact, it is a common symptom of countless skin conditions. To determine its cause, you must first determine if the dryness is consistent or if it comes and goes. If it's the latter, can you match its onset with any new scenarios? For example, periodic dryness may be caused by:

SEASONAL CHANGES

Those who live in seasonally cold climates experience skin dryness when the mercury drops, due to a lack of humidity in the air.

USE OF A NEW SKINCARE PRODUCT

Many skincare products contain ingredients that strip away the oily layer that sits atop skin. This layer is key in that it keeps moisture within the skin. When it is removed by the use of a harsh cleanser or alcohol-containing product, the skin becomes prone to dryness.

ENVIRONMENTAL FACTORS

After extensive air travel, many individuals experience skin dryness. This is due to the lack of humidity within the cabins of planes.

SMOKING

Smokers and those regularly exposed to secondhand smoke often complain of dry skin. This is believed to be due to two primary factors. First, cigarette smoke contains thousands of chemicals that encourage oxidation. As you'll recall from chapter 3, oxidation triggers free radical production, which inflicts damage upon the cells of the body, including skin cells. This damage may lead to the drying and cracking of the skin. Additionally, smoking reduces the body's stores of vitamin A. Among the vital tasks of vitamin A are to encourage skin elasticity and regulate the activity of the sebaceous glands, which secrete sebum (oil). When inadequate amounts are present in the body, skin dryness results.

MEDICATIONS

Dry skin is a side effect of a number of commonly prescribed drugs. Among them are statins (cholesterol lowering drugs), diurectics (also called "water pills"), anti-cholinergics (often used for gastrointestinal disorders), and several of the drugs used in chemotherapy. Skin dryness is also an expected side effect of many acne prescriptions, including Accutane.

If your skin dryness is caused by a medication, consult with your doctor about alternative prescriptions that may be available.

MEDICAL CONDITIONS

Skin dryness is a symptom of a number of common diseases and conditions. Some of these include eczema, psoriasis, dermatitis, diabetes, vitamin deficiency (particularly vitamin A), thyroid disorders, anorexia nervosa, and even pregnancy. If you have not been currently diagnosed with one of these conditions and have ruled out all other causes of skin dryness, it's recommended you see your doctor to determine if there is a medical connection.

RISKS

While dry skin is uncomfortable, the real issue is the damage that can ensue if it is left untreated. Persistent dryness can lead to cracking. Given that skin is our body's first line of defense against the outside world, when it is compromised, bacteria are given the opportunity to enter the body. This, in turn, may lead to infection and disease.

MYTHS

Contrary to popular belief, adding water to the skin will not increase its moisture content. You'll recall this is one of the "common myths" we reviewed in chapter 1. Simply put, skin can't absorb water. In fact, applying water to the skin can cause the opposite effect and actually exacerbate dryness.

There's another variation on this myth that is also often recommended by licensed skincare professionals: Apply lotion and moisturizers after showering when skin is still damp to lock in moisture. Again, given that skin can't absorb water, this technique will provide no benefit.

SOLUTIONS

There are a number of key practices that can improve dry skin. These include:

Utilize a moisturizer rich in humectants.

Humectants are the key component of an effective moisturizer. Rather than applying moisture to the skin, they help the skin to hold in its existing water content. They're further beneficial in that they improve the pliability of the skin.

Often, humectant-rich moisturizers are marketed as "night moisturizers." This is because they are heavier and, therefore, most convenient for nighttime wear when makeup isn't applied over the top. However, for those suffering from dry skin, night moisturizers are appropriate for daytime use, as well.

Run a humidifier in your home.

Especially for those suffering from dry skin due to a lack of humidity in their environment, as is the case in cold weather climates or for those who spend a good deal of time in air conditioning, use of a humidifier will bring some relief.

Avoid the use of irritating product ingredients.

While it's often hard to know specifically which ingredients may be causing dry skin, it's best to generally avoid those that encourage its development or make existing cases even worse. Ingredients to avoid include sodium lauryl sulfate, a detergent commonly found in cleansers and shampoos that is irritating to many individuals and encourages dry skin; alcohol, which is found in some toners and astringents and strips the skin of its protective oil layer while encouraging inflammation; and excessive fragrances. Many individuals have allergic reactions to the fragrances present in skincare products. These allergies manifest themselves in redness, itchiness, bumps, and dry patches.

Protect the skin from the sun when outdoors.
This rule doesn't apply just to seasonal extremes like sunny days or cold winters. Year-round, sunscreen should be applied before even stepping out of the house. Seasonal-appropriate coverings should also be used to protect skin from sun, wind, and cold.

Limit time spent in the shower.
Long, hot showers or baths thin the skin's lipid layer. Add to this the use of body washes or soaps, however, and you have a recipe for disaster. Instead, limit the amount of time in the shower, turn down the water temperature, and be sure to use products that utilize gentle cleansers.

Exfoliate.
Exfoliation is key to the improvement of dry skin. Proper daily chemical exfoliation removes the layer of dead cells that sits on top of the skin, revealing the newer cells beneath. Once proper exfoliation has been achieved, moisturizers become more effective. (See chapter 3 for more on exfoliation.)

Compliance is key.

Of course, each of these steps can bring about a temporary improvement in skin. But the only way to truly beat the condition is by making these practices a habit.

FINE LINES/WRINKLES

In chapter 2 we talked about the various factors that cause skin damage. Among them is chronological aging, of which fine lines and wrinkles are a hallmark. Starting in one's mid-twenties, fine lines begin appearing around the periphery of the eyes. These lines become more pronounced until, in the following decades, they deepen to become wrinkles.

While fine lines and wrinkles are, indeed, associated with aging, they are actually secondary effects caused by changes that occur within the skin. As we age, the skin's repair mechanisms begin to function less effectively. This gives the skin an overall thinned appearance and reduces its ability to hold moisture, which results in dryness. These factors, together, result in wrinkles. As if that isn't bad enough, skin cells are not shed as easily as we age, nor are they renewed as vigorously as they once were. This buildup of dead skin cells can give the skin a rough texture and accentuates the presence of wrinkles. And, because collagen and elastin levels are diminished, the structure of the skin becomes compromised, further accentuating wrinkles and giving the skin a saggy appearance.

Although this short overview of the skin's aging process may paint a dismal picture, it really is a worst-case scenario. If the skin fails to receive proper care as it ages, these challenges will only result in more pronounced lines and wrinkles. Conversely, proper care will minimize the signs of aged skin.

Each year, consumers spend more than $1 billion on wrinkle creams in the hopes they'll eliminate any lines that are present on their face. I, therefore, want to instill in you a good dose of reality. <u>Most lines and wrinkles cannot be erased.</u> Rather, we can take care of the causes of wrinkles, including dryness, stress, and dead skin buildup, which will minimize their presence.

Beyond the chronological causes outlined above, fine lines and wrinkles are also caused by:

EXPOSURE TO CIGARETTE SMOKE

Cigarette smoke contains thousands of chemicals, some of which cause collagen and elastin to break down, resulting in sagging skin. Additionally, nicotine causes blood vessels to constrict, which reduces the amount of oxygen and nutrients that can reach the skin.

EXCESS SUN EXPOSURE

Those who have spent years worshipping the sun will find that the beauty of bronzed skin gives way to wrinkles and a leathery appearance as they age. This is because sun exposure breaks down collagen and elastin, and damages the DNA of skin cells.

STRESS

As we worry, our body produces cortisol, a hormone that helps the body to prepare for "fight or flight." But while cortisol is beneficial in helping us prepare for danger, it inhibits the production of collagen.

MYTHS

As stated, consumers put far too much hope into the beautifully packaged jars of "wrinkle cream" sold at drugstores and department stores. In reality, skincare products are limited in what they can do to address fine lines and wrinkles, since they rarely reach far enough into the skin's layers to be effective.

The one caveat to this is the use of chemical exfoliants. Through the daily use of an effective exfoliation product, the keratin layer of dead skin cells can be removed. This minimizes the appearance of fine lines. (For more on proper exfoliation, see chapter 3.)

SOLUTIONS

Key practices to improve fine lines and wrinkles include:

1. Utilize an effective, daily exfoliation product to prevent the keratin layer from thickening. This practice will keep the dermis layer, the factory of the skin where collagen and elastin are produced, functioning optimally.

2. Avoid skin dryness. Use a high quality moisturizer and be sure to give your body proper nutrition. Also, be sure to take the appropriate steps to protect your skin from the elements.

While topical skincare products are limited in what they can do to address fine lines and wrinkles, a number of cosmetic procedures exist that can significantly reduce the number of wrinkles present on skin or eliminate them entirely. (More detailed explanations of each procedure can be found in chapter 2.) These include:

> *Laser resurfacing*
> *Microdermabrasion*
> *Chemical peel*
> *Thermage®*
> *Fraxel®*
> *Fillers*
> *Botox®*
> *Face lift*

PREVENTION

While wrinkles caused by the natural aging process can't be prevented, those due to environmental factors certainly can. For that reason, it's essential that sunscreen be used daily, year-round.

HYERPIGMENTATION

The correct term for areas of darkened skin is *hyperpigmentation*, yet many still refer to it as "age spots" or "liver spots." These nicknames are misleading, as hyperpigmentation is not a natural part of aging, nor is it associated in any way with the liver. Rather, hyperpigmentation occurs when certain skin cells are encouraged to release an excess of melanin (skin pigment). Reasons include:

SUN EXPOSURE

This is the most common cause of hyperpigmentation. Because of this, hyperpigmentation is often seen on the face, hands, and chest, as these are the areas most likely to experience excessive sun exposure. Because sun damage is cumulative, hyperpigmentation worsens with age. This is where the idea of "age spots" stems from.

HORMONAL CHANGES

When the body undergoes extended periods of hormonal changes, such as pregnancy or as happens with the use of birth control pills, hyperpigmentation may result. In the case of pregnancy, hyperpigmentation is called "chloasma" or is referred to by its nickname, "the mask of pregnancy." This is because chloasma commonly appears on the face, around the eyes. Following the end of pregnancy or the cessation of use of birth control pills, hyperpigmentation usually disappears, albeit slowly.

INFLAMMATION

After the skin has suffered an inflammatory wound, a type of hyperpigmentation referred to as "post-inflammatory hyperpigmentation" is commonly left behind. You may notice this type of hyperpigmentation after an acne lesion has cleared, following healing of a burn, or even after some cosmetic procedures, including chemical peels, laser resurfacing, or microdermabrasion.

MEDICAL CONDITIONS

Certain medical conditions increase the potential for hyperpigmentation. Among these are celiac disease and Addison's disease. If you suffer from a medical condition and are noticing areas of hyperpigmentation, it's important to bring the symptom to your physician's attention.

MYTHS

Areas of hyperpigmentation are often mistaken as a sign of skin cancer. Actually, the two are unrelated but certainly can coexist. Hyperpigmentation by itself may not be harmful to one's overall well-being. Rather, these areas may be simply an aesthetic concern.

SOLUTIONS

Hyperpigmentation can often be addressed via the use of a topical cream that includes skin-lightening agents, such as hydroquinone, kojic acid, and azelaic acid.

To keep hyperpigmentation under control, the best option is to utilize an effective daily exfoliant. This removes the keratin layer of dead skin cells and effectively reduces the potential for excess pigmentation.

Cosmetic procedures may be utilized for areas of significant hyperpigmentation. However, it is important to note that these treatments may also *cause* the issue. Of course, that symptom will diminish or disappear over time, but it is still a side effect you should discuss with the licensed expert conducting the procedure.

Cosmetic procedures for hyperpigmentation include:

> *Intensed Pulse Light (IPL) Therapy*
> *Fraxel®*
> *Chemical peel conducted with a bleaching agent*
> *Microdermabrasion*
> *Dermabrasion*
> *Laser resurfacing*

LARGE PORES

Large pores can be found anywhere on the face, but they most often appear on the nose and cheeks. Causes of large pores include:

OILY SKIN

People with oily skin, caused most often by overactive sebaceous glands that produce excess sebum (the skin's natural oil), are likely to have enlarged pores. This is because excess oil often results in clogged hair follicles. When the follicle is clogged, it dilates and, thus, results in a wider pore opening.

AGE

As we age, skin becomes drier and less elastic. This causes the pores to appear larger.

EXCESS SUN EXPOSURE

Sun damage causes the breakdown of collagen and elastin in our skin. Thus, people with excess sun damage will often notice that pores appear larger.

THICKENED KERATIN LAYER

When dead skin cells build up on the skin, the appearance of pores is magnified.

MYTHS

I often see "how to" articles about ways to reduce the size of your pores. Most often, these methods include the use of facial masks and creams. Unfortunately, there is no way to shrink the size of pores. Rather, we can minimize their appearance by ensuring hair follicles remain free of buildup.

SOLUTIONS

Exfoliation

My number one recommendation for minimizing the appearance of large pores is to—you guessed it—exfoliate daily with an effective product. This ensures the pores are kept free of the dirt, bacteria, and dead skin cells that build up in the hair follicle.

Cosmetic Procedures

Cosmetic procedures may also be utilized to minimize large pores. The most useful will be those that provide the skin with exfoliation, including *microdermabrasion* and *chemical peels*. However, I look at these treatments as a secondary approach after several months of regular at-home exfoliation.

OILINESS

As I mentioned, oily skin is most often caused by overactive sebaceous glands that produce excess sebum, the skin's natural oil. Sebum is beneficial in that it helps to lubricate and moisturize the hair and skin. Because dry skin is one of the factors that causes skin to look particularly "aged," those who produce excess sebum often benefit from a more youthful appearance as they get older. The downside, of course, is that oily skin is often accompanied by acne (see chapter 7) and the shine it imparts on the skin is often hard to control.

Causes of oily skin include genetics and hormone levels. Therefore, women may find their skin to be oilier during menstruation or pregnancy. Another group affected is teenagers, as puberty causes a surge in hormone production.

MYTHS

Among the treatments often touted for excess oiliness is the use of a powerful cleansing agent or astringent. Actually, this method strips the skin of its oils and can cause inflammation, which leads to the production of even more oil (this is one of the methods the body uses to respond to inflammation).

It has been recommended that sun exposure can help to "dry" the skin. While time spent in the sun can temporarily dry the skin, this method not only puts the individual at risk of skin damage, it also may lead to an increase in oil production.

SOLUTIONS

To get oily skin under control, a proper skincare regimen is key (see chapter 3 for my recommended approach). However, be sure to utilize skincare products specially formulated for oily skin. As for makeup, choose non-comedogenic and oil-free products.

Additionally, daily exfoliation with an effective formulation is beneficial in that it keeps sebum production under control and reduces the potential for inflammation.

Finally, your physician may make the determination that a prescribed solution is an effective treatment. In that case, retinoids, such as tretinoin, may be utilized.

REDNESS

"Redness" is a term that may describe two separate types of concerns. The one referred to here is characterized by a persistent red hue and is often accompanied by dryness or itching. A second type of redness is more commonly referred to as "flushing," which is temporary and may be related to a physiological condition.

Persistent skin redness is most often a telltale sign of inflammation, which can have numerous causes. Among them is irritation from an external environmental stimulus, an allergic reaction due to the application of a particular product or ingredient to the skin, or a medical condition, including rosacea or eczema.

Often, skin that suffers from redness is described as "sensitive skin." But, as mentioned in chapter 3, those symptoms considered hallmarks of sensitive skin are most often simply indicators of unhealthy skin. And in those instances, a proper skincare regimen coupled with a healthy diet can bring the biology of the skin back into balance.

SOLUTIONS

The key to eliminating redness is to first eliminate inflammation. However, because redness can be an indicator of a serious issue, such as a skin disorder, I recommend first seeking medical treatment if the condition has persisted for an extended period of time.

Once a medical condition has been ruled out, the following recommendations may be pursued:

AVOID INGREDIENTS THAT ARE KNOWN IRRITANTS.

This may include skincare products that include alcohol, powerful cleansing agents, or abrasive elements, as in the case of facial scrubs. These ingredients encourage inflammation.

IMPLEMENT AN EFFECTIVE SKINCARE REGIMEN.

See chapter 3 for my recommended skincare regimen, intended to meet the skin's basic needs.

WITHIN THE SKINCARE REGIMEN, SELECT PRODUCTS WITH INGREDIENTS PROVEN TO DIMINISH INFLAMMATION.

These ingredients may include aloe vera, niacinamide, and bisabolol.

EXFOLIATE REGULARLY WITH AN EFFECTIVE FORMULATION.

While daily exfoliation may first encourage greater redness, it will eventually eliminate dead skin cell buildup and encourage the production of collagen. This helps to eliminate symptoms of sensitive skin and get the skin back in balance.

PROTECT SKIN FROM HARSH ENVIRONMENTAL CONDITIONS.

Because redness is exacerbated by excess sun exposure and the effects of cold weather, it is highly advised that sunscreen be used daily and protective gear be worn when venturing outdoors.

ROUGH SKIN TEXTURE

Rough skin texture most often occurs as the skin ages and cellular turnover, as well as the rate at which collagen and elastin are produced, slows down. The condition can also, however, be due to a build up of dead skin cells and skin dryness.

Changes in skin texture may also be attributed to various medical conditions. For example, it is a symptom of skin disorders like rosacea, psoriasis, and eczema.

SOLUTIONS

The best method for alleviating rough skin texture is to begin exfoliating the skin daily with an effective formulation. This method will remove the keratin layer and encourage the production of collagen and elastin.

Other solutions for rough skin texture include:

IMPLEMENT A SKINCARE REGIMEN THAT SATISFIES THE SKIN'S BASIC NEEDS.

See chapter 3 for my recommended approach. This regimen must include the use of a moisturizer with the proper concentration of humectants.

Consider cosmetic procedures, including *laser skin resurfacing, chemical peels,* and exfoliation treatments like *microdermabrasion.*

UNDEREYE CIRCLES

Causes of the darkened circles under the eyes include an excess of skin pigment and the presence of dilated blood vessels. Undereye circles are considered a hereditary condition in that some individuals are just more predisposed to the issue. However, it may appear more pronounced in those with fair skin, through which blood vessels are more apparent. Additional factors include:

AGING

As we age, our skin thins due to a breakdown of collagen and slowing of its production. This thin skin allows the blood vessels below the surface to become increasingly apparent while giving the area a hollow appearance.

ALLERGIES OR NASAL CONGESTION

Congestion causes blood vessels below the skin to pool.

SMOKING

As outlined in chapter 2, smoking contributes to thin skin.

SUN EXPOSURE.

Especially in those with darker skin complexions, sun exposure may cause the pigment under the eyes to darken.

MYTHS

Fatigue and lack of sleep are commonly blamed for under-eye circles. While fatigue can cause a pale complexion that makes shadows more obvious in the under-eye area, it is not a direct cause of the issue.

SOLUTIONS

The appearance of dark undereye circles may be improved through the daily use of an effective exfoliant, as these products will help to thicken the dermis layer of the skin. Other solutions require in-office procedures:

LASER RESURFACING

This treatment is helpful when undereye circles are caused by excess pigment cells, as is the case for those with darker skin complexions.

FILLERS

The use of fillers help to thicken the area under the eyes, thus masking the presence of blood vessels.

> *Additionally, a recent Japanese study has shown some initial success in treating undereye circles with a formulation of vitamins C, E, and K along with retinol.*[12]

While this chapter outlined various treatment protocols for common skin concerns, it's important to note that this information cannot suffice for proper medical assistance. If your skin concern is persistent or severe, it's essential that you seek medical assistance from a dermatologist, plastic surgeon, or general physician.

7

ACNE

Acne's prevalence in our society is such that I felt it deserving of its own chapter. After all, it is estimated that, at any given time, forty to fifty million Americans are affected by the symptoms of acne.[13] While adolescents and young adults are most affected—a whopping 75 to 85 percent of them experience the condition—for 3 to 12 percent of the population, it persists into middle age.[14]

It should come as no surprise, then, that acne is the most common skin ailment treated by physicians. An inflammatory condition of the hair follicle, acne can result in pustules, pimples, and cysts on the skin, while persistent symptoms can lead to long-term scarring. Beyond scars of the cosmetic variety, however, acne can also cause scarring of the emotional kind. Sufferers often experience depression and anxiety, embarrassment, and social inhibition. In fact, a recent survey of British teenagers found that 39% said acne stopped them from making friends.[15] It is, therefore, obvious that treatment of acne is not just important from an aesthetic perspective—it's often key to the overall well-being of the individual suffering its symptoms.

If you count yourself among the millions who suffer from acne, chances are you've been fighting the symptoms your entire life. Acne is a chronic condition, meaning the disease is long lasting and has a propensity to recur after symptom-free periods. These factors contribute to the challenge of finding the proper treatment protocol. To that point, consumers on the quest for an acne "cure" spend billions annually on prescription and over-the-counter drugs. Yet, despite the plethora of products developed to eliminate acne symptoms, few do so successfully. Why? Because, most often, each of these products exist to address acne symptoms rather than its multiple causes. Unless each factor that causes acne is successfully addressed, acne symptoms will recur again and again.

ACNE CAUSES

For those who suffer from acne, the skin's natural rhythm of oil production and sloughing of dead skin cells is not in balance as it is for those with healthy skin. Four principle factors have been identified as causing acne:

ABNORMALLY STICKY CELLS ("FOLLICULAR KERATINIZATION")

Acne sufferers tend to have excessively "sticky" skin cells. Because of this, dead skin cells do not shed as they should and, instead, plug hair follicles (at the skin's surface, the follicle opening is called a "pore"). Attached to the hair follicles are sebaceous glands, which produce sebum, the skin's natural oil. Given that hair follicles are the "tunnel" through which sebum travels to the surface of the skin, you can understand that a blocked hair follicle causes sebum to build up.

EXCESS SEBUM PRODUCTION.

Many acne sufferers have overactive sebaceous glands that produce far more sebum than is needed by the skin. Sebaceous glands are prompted to produce oil by androgenic hormones such as testosterone and androsterone, which are affiliated with the development of masculine characteristics but are present in both males and females. When hormones change or surge, such as during adolescence, pregnancy, menstruation, or in times of stress, sebum production may increase. In some individuals, however, excess sebum production is simply a hereditary factor.

BACTERIA

Present on the skin of all adult humans is Propionibacterium, or P. acnes, the bacteria that is responsible for acne.

Because P. acnes live on fatty acids found in sebum, those individuals with excessive sebum production may also have higher than normal levels of acne bacteria on their skin. When a hair follicle becomes blocked, the buildup of sebum and dead skin cells creates the ideal environment for P. acnes. Therefore, the bacteria begins to grow within the follicle itself, rather than on the surface of the skin.

INFLAMMATION

The body's inflammation response occurs whenever tissue is damaged. Characterized by redness, swelling, warmth, and pain, inflammation happens in acne when P. acnes are prevalent within hair follicles.

Yet inflammation, while a protective response of the body, also inflicts its own damage. I explain it this way: Damage to tissue is like a house fire raging out of control. The inflammation response is like the fire department that quickly arrives to put out the flames. Once the fire is out, the house may be standing, but the property has been trampled and the structure is in disarray. In the case of acne, inflammation may address some damage at the microscopic site where bacteria once were, but in the process it can produce papules, pustules, nodules, cysts, and the like.

While these four factors can individually contribute to the development of acne, most often they work together. The typical scenario is this:

The presence of abnormally sticky cells coupled with the excessive production of sebum cause a hair follicle to plug. The obstructed follicle, engorged with oil and dead skin cells, initially becomes a comedo (see below for definitions). At this point, the follicle becomes the ideal habitat for bacteria. As bacteria flourish within the hair follicle, they release proteins (enzymes) that attract white blood cells to the area, causing inflammation that results in a pustule. If the inflammation is not controlled, the condition worsens, resulting in more serious lesions.

Beyond the four main causes of acne, however, the condition may be instigated by repeated, localized friction and irritation, as is common in violinists; below normal levels of vitamin A, which is why retinoids (a form of vitamin A) are effective in the treatment of acne; certain occupational hazards; certain medications; and, possibly, food allergies.

In the case of *occupational acne*, an individual is exposed to chemicals and other irritable substances that combine with dead skin cells to block the skin's pores, resulting in acne lesions. While the incidence of occupational acne has dropped considerably in recent years, thanks to the strengthening of workplace health and safety legislations, it does still occur. Forms include oil acne, which affects those who work with grease and/or petroleum-based cutting oils; coal-tar acne, which affects those who work with creosote and other coal tar oils; and chloracne, which affects those who work with halogenated aromatic compounds.

Jobs associated with occupational acne include, but are not limited to:

> Auto and diesel truck mechanics or assembly line workers
> Fast food workers
> Construction workers, roofers, and road pavers
> Waste handling workers
> Chemical manufacturers
> Wood preservation workers

To reduce the risk of occupational acne, workers should emphasize thorough protective measures and personal hygiene, including frequent hand and face washing and the daily use of clean workplace-appropriate clothing.

MEDICATIONS

As mentioned, several medications have been shown to trigger acne outbreaks or aggravate existing cases of acne. A direct connection, however, is often difficult to prove. This is because the condition or disease that the medication is treating is often a source of stress for the individual. Because stress can cause a surge in hormones, it is often associated with the onset of acne. This leaves physicians uncertain if the medication itself is causing the acne symptoms. Therefore, if you are taking a prescription and develop or see an increase in acne, do not stop taking the medication. Rather, consult your physician to determine if an alternative treatment may be prescribed. In cases where the prescribed medication is the only viable treatment solution, it is often necessary to treat the acne instead of ceasing administration of medication. Acne may be a psychological strain, but it is generally not dangerous and will not affect your physical well-being.

Potential acne-inducing medications include:

CONTRACEPTIVES

Contraceptives are occasionally prescribed to specifically control acne. This is due to the capacity of these medications to affect the body's hormone balance, a factor with a direct link to the development of acne.

Oral contraceptives contain both estrogen and progestin hormones. While the estrogen between contraceptive brands is fairly consistent, several types of progestin may be used, with each creating a different effect. Those that are most likely to cause acne contain low amounts of estrogen and a type of progestin that increases the androgen (male hormone) levels in women. Even in this case, however, the only women to see the onset or increase of acne are those with a tendency toward androgenicity.

ANTICONVULSANTS

Prescribed for the treatment of epilepsy, other types of seizures, bipolar disorder, and some forms of depression, certain anticonvulsants, such as Dilantin, list acne as a common side effect. Lithium, which is also used to treat bipolar disorder and depression, may also contribute to acne breakouts.

CORTICOSTEROIDS

Often used to treat asthma and other chronic lung diseases, corticosteroids act as cortisol, a natural steroid produced by the body during times of intense stress. As such, corticosteroids can stimulate sebum production, a factor involved in the development of acne.

IMMUNOSUPPRESSANTS

Used to suppress the immune system of patients awaiting organ transplantation, immunosuppressants, such as Imuran, may also suppress the body's natural ability to fight bacteria, including that which causes acne.

STEROIDS

Systemic steroids are synthetic versions of the body's natural steroid, cortisol, and are often prescribed to treat skin conditions. These medications may stimulate sebum production, a factor involved in the development of acne.

Anabolic steroids, which are used and sometimes abused by athletes and body builders to increase muscle mass, increase the presence of androgenic hormones. Again, androgenic hormones stimulate the sebaceous glands to produce sebum. An excess of male hormones causes the excess production of sebum, one of the four main causes of acne.

THYROID MEDICATIONS

Used to treat individuals with low thyroid function, these medications have been shown to trigger acne. Additionally, large amounts of iodine, another substance used to help regulate thyroid function, has also been shown to cause acne breakouts.

DIET

While one's diet is not a direct factor in the development of acne, the ingredients in certain foods may cause allergic reactions in some individuals. Among those reactions may be acne breakouts. Foods with the potential to cause such reactions include:

BEER

Among the main ingredients in beer is yeast. For those with yeast allergies, beer is recognized by the body as a toxin and, depending upon the severity of the allergy, consumption may cause acne to develop. The severity of the outbreak is dependent upon the body's sensitivity to yeast.

MILK

A 2005 study showed that those who drank three or more cups of milk a day were 22 percent more likely to experience severe acne compared with those who drank less than one serving each week.[16] The study showed an even stronger correlation between acne and the consumption of skim milk, in particular. The study's author suggested that hormones and bioactive molecules present in milk are responsible for exacerbating acne.

HIGH GLYCEMIC LEVELS

Recent studies have shown that the glycemic level of foods may play a role in the development or cessation of acne. Foods with high glycemic levels, including white bread, potatoes, and most processed foods, cause a large insulin response after ingestion. This elevated level of insulin in the body triggers a "hormonal cascade" that leads to increased production of substances known to contribute to acne formation.[17] Conversely, low glycemic load diets that contain more whole grains and vegetables have been shown to reduce the presence of acne.

TYPES OF ACNE LESIONS

While most individuals consider any type of acne lesion to be a "pimple," there are actually several categories that relate to the disease:

COMEDO

Characterized by a plugged and, thereby, enlarged hair follicle, there are two types of comedones. A *closed comedo* (also called a "whitehead") is a blockage deep below the skin pore. Because it is deep, it leaves only a microscopic opening at the skin's surface, which air cannot penetrate. Because of the lack of oxygen, the dead skin cells and sebum present in the follicle do not oxidize, leaving them colorless and giving them their white appearance. An *open comedo* (also called a "blackhead") is a blockage that is close to the skin's surface. Because of its location, the pore is enlarged, allowing oxygen to reach the blockage. This oxidation coupled with the way the blockage reflects light gives the comedo a dark hue, causing it to appear brown or black.

PAPULE

Caused by inflammation, papules are round, raised red bumps that do not have a fluid or pus-filled center. They tend to be painful and, if squeezed, can become infected.

PUSTULE

Also caused by inflammation, pustules appear similar to pap-ules, with the addition of a white or yellow pus-filled cen-ter. This is the type of lesion commonly called a "pimple."

NODULE

When inflammation is allowed to worsen, the blockage within the hair follicle coupled with a bacterial invasion can cause the follicle to rupture, resulting in nodules—large, hard lumps below the skin's surface. Nodules are often painful and take weeks or even months to heal. If not properly treated, nodules can recur repeatedly at the same site and have a high propensity for scarring.

CYST

Similar to a nodule, cysts are caused by severe inflammation after a rupture in the hair follicle wall and a bacterial inva-sion. The difference is that cysts are larger and filled with pus. Again, cysts may recur at the same site if left untreated and have a tendency to leave scars. What's more, nodules and cysts can create channels between them, which makes severe acne all the more difficult to treat.

TYPES OF ACNE

To establish the proper course of treatment, skincare pro-fessionals must first determine the type of acne from which an individual is suffering. To do this, the professional thoroughly examines the skin to review the acne lesions that are present, along with the prevalence of each. Among the acne types and classifications are:

ACNE VULGARIS

This is the most common type of acne and is classified by the severity of the acne lesions.

Mild acne is characterized by the presence of comedones, including either whiteheads or blackheads or both.

Moderate acne is characterized by the presence of papules and pustules. Whiteheads and blackheads may also be visible.

Severe acne is characterized by the presence of nodules and cysts.

Severe acne has several forms. These include:

Acne Conglobata

Occurring most often in males, acne conglobata is characterized by a proliferation of comedones, pustules, and nodules. The nodules may become interconnected through channels, which causes extensive scarring. Acne conglobata is often resistant to treatment.

Acne Fulminans

This type of acne develops quite suddenly and is characterized by extensive inflammation. This inflammation isn't limited simply to acne lesions, however. Rather, it may cause pain in joints, swelling of the lymph nodes, and fever. Acne fulminans can be severe to the extent that hospitalization becomes necessary.

Gram Negative Folliculitus

Individuals who have acne vulgaris and have been treated with antibiotics for an extensive period of time may develop gram negative folliculitus. This type of acne is characterized by the presence of pustules, nodules, and cysts. In most cases, as soon as the antibiotic is discontinued, symptoms of gram negative folliculitus end.

Nodulocystic Acne

Causing significant discomfort, nodulocystic acne is characterized by the presence of numerous pus-filled cysts most often on the face, neck, and back. Nodulocystic acne has the potential to cause extensive and severe scarring.

MYTHS SURROUNDING ACNE

For years, several factors were commonly accepted as causes of acne. However, research in recent years has either disproven the correlation between these factors and acne, or failed to prove a link. Among the more prevalent *myths* relative to the causes of acne are:

CLEANLINESS

Acne is not caused by poor hygiene and cannot be remedied by excessive scrubbing or washing. In fact, doing so could actually worsen acne symptoms. Furthermore, there is no correlation between acne severity and skin bacteria numbers.

CHOCOLATE/GREASY FOODS

The notion that eating chocolate or greasy foods will cause acne has been passed down for decades; yet, no evidence exists to support this claim. The caveat to this statement is that those with milk allergies (lactose intolerance) may react to the milk found in chocolate. In this case, chocolate has the potential to cause acne as the body interprets the presence of milk as a toxin.

STRESS

The relationship between acne and stress remains controversial. Most studies do not support a direct correlation.

However, during times of stress the body produces cortisol, which can stimulate sebum production, a factor involved in the development of acne. Additionally, stress may interfere with sleep quality and general health, which may indirectly influence the development of acne symptoms.

MAKEUP

While makeup does not have the capacity to directly cause acne, some makeup products may dry out the skin, which increases its susceptibility to the condition. For this reason, it is recommended that only non-comedogenic or non-acnegenic makeup products be used.

FACIAL STEAMING

Repeated exposure to steam may worsen acne by increasing inflammation, but it does not cause it. Occasional steaming to remove comedones is acceptable.

ACNE TREATMENT

What follows are some of the over-the-counter substances, including some homeopathic ingredients, which are beneficial in the fight against acne. While none of them address all four causes of acne alone, ingredients such as these may be combined in a single formulation or within product families to offer a complete solution to not only control symptoms but to also help regulate the factors that cause the disease.

INGREDIENTS TO ADDRESS FOLLICULAR KERATINIZATION (STICKY DEAD SKIN CELLS):

Retinyl Propionate

Retinoids, a form of vitamin A, have long been used successfully in acne treatments. In fact, tretinoin, an acid form of vitamin A, is one of the most prescribed acne remedies today. In over-the-counter skincare products, retinol, the alcohol form of vitamin A, is often used. However, in some individuals it is irritating to the skin.

Retinyl propionate, a storage form of vitamin A that concentrates in the epidermis, is less irritating, and it's been found beneficial in improving acne. For example, a recent study intended to show retinyl propionate's effects on sun-damaged skin instead demonstrated a near complete reduction in acne among the study participants who suffered from the disease.[18]

Glycolic Acid

Glycolic acid is the smallest, molecularly, of all the alpha hydroxy acids and can, therefore, penetrate easily between cells to loosen dead skin, remove cell buildup inside the hair follicle, and open clogged pores, comedones, and other impactions in oily areas. Continued use helps keep dead skin cells from accumulating on the follicle wall, thus preventing inflammatory acne lesions. A recent study showed products with glycolic acid significantly reduced comedones, papules, and pustules and reduced the size of pores while rejuvenating skin texture.[19]

Salicylic Acid

Salicylic acid, a beta hydroxy acid, works to soften and exfoliate the dead skin of the dermis layer. By opening clogged pores, salicylic acid helps to reestablish the normal skin cell renewal cycle. Comparative studies of salicylic acid have shown it to be superior even to benzoyl peroxide in reducing the total number of acne lesions.[20]

Salicylic acid is further beneficial in the treatment of acne due to its antimicrobial properties, which kill acne bacteria.

INGREDIENTS TO ADDRESS EXCESS SEBUM PRODUCTION:

Zinc Pyrithione

An antibacterial and antifungal agent developed in the 1930s, zinc pyrithione works to stop the growth of certain bacteria on the skin, including P. acnes. Due to its ability to regulate sebum production, it is beneficial in the treatment of acne and is further used to treat scalp disorders, such as dandruff, psoriasis, and seborrheic dermatitis.

Sulfur

One of only a handful of over-the-counter acne treatments to secure FDA approval, sulfur is among the oldest medicines still in use. In the treatment of acne, it reduces oil gland activity and dissolves the skin's surface layer of dry, dead cells. Additionally, it inhibits the growth of P. acnes.

Among the research related to sulfur's use in the treatment of acne, one study demonstrated that sulfur lotion reduced acne symptoms by 83 percent after 12 weeks of treatment.[21]

Niacinamide

Also known as vitamin B3, niacinamide decreases the production of a fatty acid (triglyceride) in the sebaceous glands. Therefore, it is capable of reducing sebum excretion rates and overall sebum levels. Additionally, niacinamide acts as a potent anti-inflammatory.

Vitamin D

Acquired by the body both from the diet and by exposure to sunlight (hence its nickname of "vitamin of the sun"), vitamin D reduces the size of sebaceous glands, thereby reducing the sebum that becomes trapped in clogged pores. Evidence has suggested that acne may be caused by a vitamin D deficiency.

INGREDIENTS TO ADDRESS COLONIZATION OF P. ACNES:

Benzoyl peroxide

A potent antiseptic, benzoyl peroxide is one of the most commonly used ingredients in the treatment of acne. It is effective at eliminating P. acnes and reduces the quantity of comedones. An added bonus—benzoyl peroxide doesn't promote antibacterial resistance, as can happen with the use of prescription antibiotics.

Eucalyptus oil

The most versatile essential oil found in nature, eucalyptus oil has been used for sinus relief, sore throats, as a topical antiseptic for skin injuries, and as an inhalant for asthma and other respiratory conditions. It has proven effective in the treatment of acne due to its antiseptic properties, as well as its ability to inhibit the growth of P. acnes.[22]

Tea Tree Oil

Extracted from the leaves of the Australian Melaleuca alternafolia tree, topical application of tea tree oil helps to reduce bacteria on the skin, lessens inflammation, and generally improves the symptoms of acne. In fact, a study comparing tea tree oil to the use of benzoyl peroxide demonstrated improvements among patients in both groups, while those using tea tree oil reported fewer side effects (stinging, itching, burning, and dryness).[23]

INGREDIENTS TO ADDRESS INFLAMMATION:

Aloe vera

A plethora of research exists to demonstrate aloe vera's potent anti-inflammatory abilities. Of the more than two hundred active components in aloe, it contains salicylic acid and sterols, both of which work to inhibit inflammation. Aloe also has antimicrobial properties and is, therefore, beneficial in helping control P. acnes.

Arnica

Commonly referred to as "leopard's bane," the arnica flower has been used in homeopathic medicine for hundreds of years. Arnica features anti-inflammatory and antibacterial properties and aids in the healing of topical skin wounds.

Bisabolol

A colorless viscous oil derived from chamomile, bisabolol has anti-inflammatory properties and is effective in reducing the potential for scar formation caused by acne.

FURTHER FACTORS TO ENCOURAGE RESULTS

Of course, the appropriate recommended at-home treatment depends greatly upon the severity of acne symptoms. If you suffer from advanced symptoms, such as cysts, a visit to your physician is necessary, as prescribed medicines, such as antibiotics or steroids, may be the most effective course of action.

Acne is a chronic problem and, as such, controlling it requires patience. For many, this process takes months or even years. In the case of acne, I always recommend the first step in treatment be a consultation with a licensed skincare expert, including a dermatologist or esthetician. As noted earlier, they can examine your acne symptoms to determine the type of acne from which you're suffering. This will result in a much more targeted treatment protocol.

Beyond the use of a targeted acne treatment product or prescription, other points to keep in mind to accelerate healing include:

WHILE DIET IS NOT A DIRECT CAUSE OF ACNE, POOR NUTRITION CAN EXACERBATE ACNE CONDITIONS.

It's beneficial to fill the bulk of your diet with fresh fruits and vegetables, whole grains, and beans, as these foods are good sources of antioxidants. Additionally, it may be helpful to avoid foods with high glycemic levels, such as white bread and potatoes, as they cause a rapid surge in blood sugar, which may lead to the development of acne.

AVOID THE USE OF ALL OTHER ACNE TREATMENTS BEYOND THOSE THAT HAVE BEEN RECOMMENDED BY YOUR SKINCARE PROFESSIONAL.

Most acne sufferers have a surplus of over-the-counter acne treatment products at home. It's important, however, to ensure you discontinue the use of anything outside the regimen that has been recommended or prescribed to you. This allows your skincare professional to know if the current treatment is effective or if modifications should be made. Additionally, many drugstore acne treatments contain abrasive ingredients that could cause inflammation, thereby exacerbating acne conditions.

UTILIZE ONLY NON-COMEDOGENIC MAKEUP.

Again, makeup isn't a direct cause of acne, but certain products may exacerbate the conditions that do cause acne. Use of non-comedogenic makeup is a precautionary step.

DO NOT TRY TO "POP" ACNE LESIONS.

Extractions must be left to a skincare professional to avoid further inflammation and the spread of acne symptoms.

ACNE SCARS

When the skin experiences an injury, such as an acne lesion, the body sends white blood cells and a host of inflammatory mediator molecules to the site to begin repairing the tissue and fighting infection. However, following the repair of damaged tissue, these white blood cells and inflammatory mediators may stay at the site for a long period of time, resulting in the formation of fibrous scar tissue. Remember my analogy about the fire department leaving a mess on your property after putting out the flames?

Not all individuals who suffer from acne are left with scars, however. The reasons why some are more scar-prone than others are not well understood. Those who do experience them, however, have them in one of two forms—either depressed marks on the skin's surface or raised, thickened areas. While some will see these scars remain for a lifetime, others may notice the scars diminish in appearance with the passing of time. Again, the reasons for this difference between individuals is not well understood.

Depressed scars occur because of a loss of tissue. There are several subcategories of depressed scars, including:

Depressed fibrotic scars, which are usually large and characterized by sharp edges with steep sides and a firm base.

Soft scars, which are soft to the touch and can be either deep or located at the skin's surface. These types of scars are usually small and are characterized by soft edges. They may be either circular or elongated.

Ice-pick scars, which most often occur on the cheek. They are most often small with a somewhat jagged edge and steep sides.

Atrophic macules are soft and often feature a wrinkled base. They may be bluish in appearance due to the blood vessels lying beneath them. Generally small when they appear on the face, these scars may be larger on other areas of the body. Over time they may change from a bluish color to ivory in light-skinned individuals.

Hypertrophic scars are raised scars that occur due to an excess of collagen, which is produced in response to the acne lesion. This excess collagen is heaped into fibrous piles, resulting in a firm, smooth, and irregularly shaped scar that typically is one to two millimeters in width. These types of scars often diminish over time.

Hypertrophic scars are often confused with *keloids*, a less common type of raised scar. Unlike those of the hypertrophic variety, keloid scars tend to grow beyond the original site of injury and do not diminish over time. They are more common in individuals with darker skin.

Another type of hypertrophic scar is *follicular macular atrophy* or *perifollicular elastosis*. This type of scar is more often to occur on the chest or back and features small, white, soft lesions that are just barely raised above the skin's surface. In fact, this type of scar may resemble a whitehead. They tend to last for months to years but eventually do diminish.

The final category of acne scars is that of *macules* or *pseudoscars*. Generally flat, reddish spots that are caused by inflammatory acne lesions, macules "mark the spot" where a lesion once was and remain for six months or more. They do, however, eventually disappear, leaving no trace.

TREATMENT OF ACNE SCARS

For those suffering from mild acne, most scarring is temporary, and all traces of acne lesions are undetectable within months to years of getting the condition under control. For those with more severe acne or acne that has been uncontrolled for a significant amount of time, however, scarring can be permanent unless cosmetic or surgical intervention is pursued. The good news is that numerous treatment options exist for most types of scarring. Some of the more popular options recommended by skincare professionals and plastic surgeons are outlined below. A more thorough overview of each treatment may be found in chapter 2.

Fillers may be injected under a raised scar to elevate it, thus minimizing its presence. Among the fillers that may be used are fat, collagen, or hyaluronic acid.

Microdermabrasion removes only the surface cells of the skin so no additional wound is created. Multiple procedures are often necessary, but scars, especially those of the hypertrophic variety, will be significantly improved after a single session.

Dermabrasion is among the most effective treatments for acne scars. Not only is the surface skin removed, but the contour of scars is also altered. Those scars located at the skin's surface may be completely eliminated, while the depth of other scars may be reduced. It does not work for all types of scars, however. It may make ice-pick scars more noticeable if they are wider under the skin than at the surface.

Laser Treatment may be used to modify the appearance of scars, while redness surrounding healed acne lesions may be reduced.

Skin Surgery may be effective on more troublesome scars. For example, ice pick scars may be removed by "punch" excision.

In this procedure, each scar is completely cut out of the skin and a suture is used to repair the remaining hole. Depressed scars may be treated via subcision, a technique in which a surgical probe is used to lift the scar tissue away from the skin.

Skin Grafting may be necessary under certain conditions, such as when microdermabrasion has exposed "tunnels" (called sinus tracts) below the skin, which are created due to inflammation. Skin grafting is, therefore, used to close the defect.

ACNE TREATMENT AND PREGNANCY

Because elevated hormone levels during pregnancy bring about a number of skin changes, acne among them, it is worthwhile to address this special circumstance. While non-pregnant women may benefit from prescription medications to treat acne, including tretinoin and isotretinoin or antibiotics such as tetracycline, erythromycin, and doxycycline, most of these medications are inappropriate for use by those who are pregnant or trying to conceive. Additionally, some over-the-counter acne treatment ingredients should be avoided during pregnancy, such as salicylic acid.

If you are within this group and are seeking treatment for acne, be sure to advise your physician so an alternative acne treatment protocol may be utilized.

8

THE EFFECTS OF CANCER TREATMENT ON THE SKIN

Throughout my years in practice I've worked often with those who are undergoing, or have recently undergone, treatment for various cancers. Beyond reconstruction following breast cancer, the most common reason these individuals come to me is to address the skin issues that result from treatment. After all, of the numerous side effects associated with radiation therapy, chemotherapy, and other cancer treatments, those that affect the skin are most common. Despite this, the topic of proper skincare in conjunction with cancer treatment is one that is grossly overlooked, in my opinion. Given that an estimated 1.5 million Americans are diagnosed with cancer each year, the need for information on the subject is great.

RADIATION THERAPY

Those who've never experienced cancer may not be aware of the damaging effects these therapies have on the skin. Yet, when you consider that the role of cancer treatment is to ravage cancer cells, you begin to understand the impact they have on non-cancerous cells as well, including healthy skin cells. In the case of radiation therapy, the skin is a direct participant in the treatment, as radiation beams pass through its surface to reach the site of cancer. This inhibits the ability of skin cells to regenerate. For this reason, as many as 95% of cancer patients treated with radiation therapy will experience a skin reaction.[24]

Commonly, individuals undergoing radiation therapy experience general skin irritation characterized by redness; itching; sensitivity or pain, similar to sunburn; and even peeling and blistering. In fact, this reaction is so common that it has been given the name *radiation dermatitis*. Symptoms of radiation dermatitis range from mild to severe and are often determined by the dose and frequency of treatment. While symptoms begin to lessen two to four weeks following therapy, for those undergoing regular treatment, radiation dermatitis is often an everyday part of the fight against cancer.

Radiation therapy is also associated with *hyperpigmentation*. Individuals with light skin tones may notice their skin becoming reddened or taking on a tanned appearance, while darker skin tones will become increasingly darkened or ashen. Freckles and moles will darken as well. Generally, hyperpigmentation occurs specifically in those areas of the skin exposed to radiation beams.

Long term radiation therapy may result in *photosensitivity*, that is, sensitivity to the sun's rays, especially at the site(s) of treatment. This puts cancer patients at an increased risk of developing skin cancer—not only during treatment, but beyond as well.

In extreme cases, patients undergoing radiation therapy may experience *radiation burn*. Evidenced by painful open sores and blisters, radiation burn mimics a chemical burn more than a sunburn. Radiation burns cause skin damage that is significant and may be visible long after cancer treatment has ceased. Doctors will generally address radiation burn and other skin complications related to radiation therapy with the use of a topical anti-inflammatory both during and after treatment.

CHEMOTHERAPY

Skin changes associated with chemotherapy are similar to that of radiation therapy. But, whereas in radiation therapy issues are generally isolated to the area(s) exposed to radiation beams, in chemotherapy, reactions in the skin tend to be systemic, as the treatment involves the delivery of cancer-fighting drugs to the body's circulatory system.

The severity of side effects is, of course, related to the dosage of chemotherapy drugs utilized and the method of delivery. Drugs delivered intravenously or via injection typically have a higher likelihood of causing changes in the skin than those delivered orally.

Among the common side effects of chemotherapy drugs are the following:

Rashes, including *acneiform*, which mimics the app-earance of acne, but, unlike acne, pustules contain no bacteria. Drugs likely to cause rashes include erlotinib and gefitinib.

Overall skin dryness. This reaction is common in drugs such as fluorouracil and cetuximab.

Hyperpigmentation, which may be seen as blotches throughout the body or specifically along the body's venous pathways. Hyperpigmentation commonly ac-companies drugs such as daunorubicin, busulfan, and bleomycin.

Photosensitivity causes skin to burn more easily. Among the drugs that cause this reaction are methotrexate and vinblastine.

TREATMENT OF SKIN DURING AND AFTER CANCER

While the goal of those experiencing skin complications due to cancer treatment may be to eliminate the issue at hand, the larger intention should be to, instead, optimize the condition of the skin overall to best minimize the impact of skin reactions. Keep in mind, however, that the sensitive immune system of cancer patients must be taken into consideration when determining the steps that are taken to improve the skin and the products that are used. This is especially true for those who are undergoing chemotherapy, which decreases white blood cell counts, thus compromising the immune system.

While most skin complications subside upon the completion of cancer treatment, some skin issues may remain for months or even years. More concerning, still, is the reality that some skin damage will be permanent. In these instances, a consultation with a skincare professional, such as a plastic surgeon or dermatologist, may be the most appropriate course of action.

SEEK OUT GENTLE INGREDIENTS AND FORMULATIONS.

It is vital that the products used on the skin of cancer patients be gentle. For that reason, no harsh soaps should be used. Additionally, be sure to investigate product labels for evidence of harsh ingredients, such as alcohol, acetone, camphor, sodium lauryl sulfate, abrasives, or excess fragrance.

ENSURE EFFECTIVE MOISTURIZATION.

Because dry skin is a common annoyance for those undergoing cancer treatment, it's important to increase the use of moisturizers to avoid further complication. If left untreated, dryness may worsen, leading to cracking of the skin. Skin is our body's first line of defense against the outside world—thus, when it becomes cracked, bacteria may be given opportunity to enter the body and could lead to infection and further complications.

Look for products that are rich in humectants, as they help the skin hold in its existing water content and improve its pliability. Generally, the more humectant-rich the moisturizer, the heavier it may be. These products are often marketed as "night moisturizers."

More information about combating dry skin may be found in chapter 6.

ONLY THE ESSENTIAL STEPS.

Throughout the pages of this book you've read the benefits of a four-step skincare regimen that cleanses, exfoliates, moisturizes, and protects the skin. For those undergoing cancer treatment, however, I advise against the use of exfoliation products.

While use of an effective daily exfoliant can certainly improve the health of the skin, those with a weakened immune system are limited in their body's ability to tolerate the acids utilized in such products. Additionally, because the body may not be able to properly generate new collagen, the benefits to this step are restricted somewhat.

Instead, implement the cleansing and moisturization steps both morning and night, with the application of additional moisturizer throughout the day, as needed. Use of sun protection is vital because of the increased photosensitivity common in those undergoing cancer treatments. However, if open sores or a rash are present, it's best to consult your physician about the products you may utilize. In some cases, sun protection must be garnered via the use of protective clothing rather than use of a product with SPF.

CONSIDER THE BENEFITS OF ALOE.

In chapter 5, I outlined the various reasons why aloe is a superior ingredient for use in skincare applications, including:

Aloe penetrates tissue.

Aloe acts as an anesthetic.

Aloe has microbial properties.

Aloe is an anti-inflammatory.

Aloe is proven to heal wounds.

Aloe is moisturizing.

For these reasons, as well as the fact that aloe is extremely gentle, it is an excellent substance for use in treatment of the skin of cancer patients. Much research has been done specifically on aloe's effectiveness on radiation injuries. In fact, the first documented aloe research dates back to 1935 when Collins and Collins found aloe to be beneficial in the treatment of radiation dermatitis. In my own practice, I regularly use organic, pharmaceutical-grade aloe when treating radiation wounds. Time and time again, this practice has allowed me to help my patients avoid scarring while accelerating healing time. (On a side note, a 2009 study showed that oral delivery of aloe in conjunction with chemotherapy increased the efficacy of treatment in terms of tumor regression and survival time.)[25]

That's not to say you should buy an aloe plant for treatment of skin issues attributed to cancer treatment. As I outlined in chapter 5, there's a difference between the purified and concentrated form of aloe that is used in medical practice and that which is found in the raw stalk of the aloe houseplant. Rather, it is beneficial to utilize skincare products that utilize a high grade of aloe in high concentrations. Look for products that list pharmaceutical-grade aloe as one of the first ingredients. But, as mentioned earlier, but sure to avoid these products if they utilize harsh ingredients.

OPTIMIZE YOUR DIET.

In chapter 3, I address some of the dietary changes that are needed to improve the health of one's skin. These suggestions promote overall good health and are, therefore, beneficial to those undergoing cancer treatment as well.

Increased consumption of foods rich in antioxidants is one of the most important dietary improvements. As the "soldiers" of our cells, antioxidants work to prevent cellular damage. There are thousands of known antioxidants, which fall into several antioxidant categories, including carotenoids, flavonoids, and polyphenols. Foods rich in antioxidants include beans and other legumes; fruits, such as berries; nuts and seeds; and a vast array of vegetables.

ONCOLOGY AESTHETICS

An emerging area of aesthetics, as evidenced by the increasing number of spas that provide such services, is that of *oncology aesthetics*. In oncology aesthetics, estheticians who are trained in techniques specific to cancer patients, provide spa treatments that encourage the release of endorphins to reduce stress and anxiety, aid in pain management, and promote healing. Intended as an integrative therapy that complements medical treatment, oncology aesthetics is further intended to improve the self-image of cancer patients.

Oncology aesthetic treatments, which may include facials, reflexology, and body wraps, utilize gentle products that are free of fragrances and other irritating ingredients, in combination with a healing touch. Additionally, an emphasis is placed on a high level of sanitation to ensure the environment isn't harmful to the individual.

Because oncology aesthetics is a new area of the field, much is yet to be learned about its benefits. However, at a minimum, such treatments may be helpful in improving the comfort level of the individual while boosting mood.

Due to the growing trend of hospitals adding complementary therapies to their offerings, issues such as the skincare needs of cancer patients may soon find that information is more readily available on the topic. In fact, some hospitals are beginning to offer oncology aesthetics in-house. In the meantime, however, it's essential for cancer patients to seek out the appropriate protocols to improve the health of their skin and, thus, enhance its ability to fight the issues that plague it during treatment. While this chapter presented some guidelines, I advise talking with your doctor about your unique skin issues and requesting referral to a dermatologist or plastic surgeon if more in-depth treatment is necessary.

FREQUENTLY ASKED QUESTIONS

I often receive e-mail from consumers who are confused about specific aspects of skincare. Some questions are so common that I'm confident they're topics of concern for many of you as well. Outlined below are some of those questions, as well as others that bring up key points about skin health. Much of the content included in the answers can be found in more detail in previous areas of the book.

If you don't see the answer you're looking for, I invite you to email me directly at DrA@Lexli.com.

GENERAL SKINCARE

Q: Is acne caused by dirt (or chocolate)?

A: Among the many factors blamed for acne, dirt and chocolate are among the two most common. Acne simply isn't caused by the presence of dirt on the skin or the consumption of chocolate. Rather, acne is caused by the clogging of pores by sloughed skin cells.

Belief in the myth that dirt causes acne has led many to overwash their skin. This practice only make matters worse by causing irritation and inflammation, which exacerbates acne.

And as for chocolate—nothing you eat can directly affect the severity of acne. Indirectly, however, certain ingredients may cause allergies, which have acne as a symptom. Additionally, unhealthy eating can lead to bad health, which can make symptoms worse.

(For more, see chapter 6.)

Q: Will my skin age in the same fashion as my mother's?

A: Genetics do play an important role in the manner in which the skin ages. However, assuming that your skin will ultimately resemble your mother's is a narrow assumption. Genetics is only one factor in skin aging. Lifestyle decisions and environmental factors, such as sun exposure and smoking, are also important determinants of skin aging.

(For more, see chapter 2.)

Q: Do moisturizers increase the moisture content of my skin?

A: Moisturizers work by *preventing* water evaporation from the skin.

Among the myths I've heard regarding moisturizers is that applying lotions or moisturizers over moist skin upon stepping out of the shower helps to trap the water and hydrate the skin. The first problem with this claim is that skin cannot absorb water. The second is that water actually encourages the skin to dry out as it evaporates.

(For more, see chapters 3 and 4.)

Q: I have combination skin. Do I require two different cleansers, two different moisturizers, etc?
A: No. Combination skin does not require special products, but it does require treating each area differently. Dry areas should be moisturized twice a day, oilier areas less often.

Q: Is it okay to use bar soap on my face?
A: This is never a good practice. Rather, I recommend the use of a pH-balanced liquid cleanser. The ingredients used to keep soaps in bar form can clog pores, contributing to breakouts. Proper cleansing sets the stage for each of the following steps in a skincare regimen.

(For more, see chapter 3.)

Q: What causes the dry patches on my face?
A: There are a number of reasons why your skin may develop dry patches, ranging from leaving makeup on the skin overnight to using the incorrect skincare products for

your skin to allergic reactions. If the patches are chronic or itchy, you may have a type of topical dermatitis that requires treatment by a physician. Some dry patches may indicate the onset of seborrheic keratosis or dermatitis. If they persist, consult your dermatologist or a plastic surgeon immediately for further evaluation of the problem. Otherwise, simply ensure you are implementing a proper skincare regimen (see chapter 3), and if the problem continues, document specifically when you are seeing the patches appear and any special circumstances that may be related to them. This will help your physician or skincare professional narrow the cause.

(For more, see chapter 6.)

Q: I want my skin to look its best, but I get confused when I listen to sales people at cosmetic counters or read the ads in my favorite magazines. How do I know what to believe and who to trust without spending a small fortune?

A: Your best choice is always a trained professional who understands skin physiology. A trained skincare professional will review your medical history, customize your treatment plan, and follow up by monitoring your treatment and progress regularly.

Q: I have oily skin and use oil-free products. However, my skin still feels oily. Why?

A: Never rely on the term "oil-free" to ensure your product features a sound formulation. Outside of oils, many "oil-free" products still contain ingredients that can clog pores, causing breakouts.

Rarely will oil-free products eliminate oily skin. Rather, you need to ensure you're implementing a proper skincare regimen (see chapter 3), one that includes exfoliation as a daily step.

Q: I'm confused. I thought water was good for your skin.

A: The ingredients included in skincare products must be listed on the packaging in order of concentration. If the first ingredient is water, stated in any manner, the product is water-based. The problem with this is the fact that the skin cannot absorb water. Furthermore, the presence of water only dilutes the other product ingredients, many of which may be beneficial.

Water is indeed beneficial to your skin when ingested. Therefore, it is important to ensure proper hydration.

SUN EXPOSURE AND PROTECTION

Q: Isn't daily sun exposure necessary for the production of vitamin D?

A: No. Vitamin D is widely available in various food products, fruits, and vegetables. Additionally, over-the-counter supplements can help the body reach its daily requirement of vitamin D. There is no reason why the sun must be relied upon as the sole source of vitamin D.

If you insist upon getting vitamin D from the sun, keep in mind that it can be produced with minimal amounts of sun exposure—such as that obtained from a short walk outdoors. However, sun exposure can negatively impact the skin. Therefore, it is recommended that sunscreen be used regularly.

Q: Won't getting a "base tan" offer protection from burning during my beach visits?

A: When exposed to the sun, skin produces melanin, which gives it the tanned appearance. Melanin produced during tanning is not as protective as the natural, genetically adaptive melanin typically produced by the skin, nor is it permanent. The act of getting a base tan causes cell damage and inflammation. Further tanning on top of that only multiplies the skin damage.

Q: Is it true that sun damage is cumulative?

A: Yes. Damage by UV light to the DNA of your cells accumulates over time. The wrinkles, fine lines, or hyperpigmentation that appear at the age of forty may very well be the result of sun exposure as a child.

EXFOLIATION

Q: How often should I exfoliate?

A: At minimum, I recommend exfoliating once per day. Depending upon the extent of skin damage, twice per day may be recommended. (Most individuals need to slowly build to this frequency.) It is essential that the exfoliation product be effective, however. To determine this, pay attention to the product's pH level. And, to ensure you won't experience burn, look for anti-inflammatory ingredients, like aloe, near the top of the ingredients list. ·

(For more, see chapter 3.)

Q: Is it true that frequent exfoliation can lead to thin skin?

A: No. If done appropriately, exfoliation can actually lead to a thickened, healthy dermis. When you exfoliate, you're encouraging the skin to produce collagen and elastin, the proteins that give the skin structure and strength.

(For more, see chapter 3.)

Q: Should exfoliation products be used around the eye area?

A: Exfoliation around the eye area can certainly be done without issue and I do recommend it. However, it is essential that care be used to ensure acid does not get in the eyes.

Q: Can regular exfoliation cause the skin to dry?

A: Yes, it can initially. For this reason, I recommend

the regular use of an effective moisturizer. Once the dermis thickens and is healthier, you may not need as much moisturizing.

Q: How do you know when the dermis has thickened?
A: As the dermis thickens, the skin will be tighter and appear healthier, with fewer signs of damage.

Q: Is it necessary to use an exfoliant when you're young? I'm twenty-five and my skin is still in good condition.
A: "Prevention" is the answer. Even at the age of twenty-five, using an exfoliant is a good idea. Helping dead skin slough off offers the opportunity for plumper, healthier skin cells to come to the surface. This helps to preserve that youthful and fresh look.

GLOSSARY

Acidic—Acidic refers to a compound or product that contains a high percentage of acid in the form of free hydrogen ions. To be acidic, it must have a pH value between 0 and 7.

Acne Conglobata—A type of acne more common in males, acne conglobata is characterized by a proliferation of comedones, pustules, and nodules. Channels may develop between the nodules, making treatment complicated. In fact, acne conglobata may be resistant to treatment.

Acne Cyst—A type of acne lesion caused by inflammation, cysts are similar to nodules in that they develop after the hair follicles rupture. Cysts are larger than nodules and are filled with pus.

Acne Fulminans—A type of acne that develops suddenly and is characterized by extensive inflammation. This inflammation may also affect the joints and cause swelling of the lymph nodes along with fever. Hospitalization often becomes necessary with this type of severe acne.

Acne Vulgaris—This is the most common type of acne. It is characterized by the presence of whiteheads, blackheads, papules, and/or pustules.

Active Skincare Agents—Ingredients that enhance cellular repair by stimulating and improving naturally occurring skin functions. Among their many abilities, active skincare agents can reflect, scatter, or block UV light, as in sunscreens; exfoliate, thus stimulating the production of collagen; lighten skin pigmentation; and prevent cellular damage, as in antioxidant formulations.

Alkaline—Another term for "basic" and the opposite of acidic, alkaline substances have a pH value between 7 and 14.

Alpha Hydroxy Acids (AHAs)—The family name for a group of naturally occurring acids often referred to as "fruit acids." The benefits attributed to these active substances include a reduction of fine lines and superficial wrinkles; a lightening of surface pigmentation; and softer, smoother, and more supple skin with improved hydration. Acids that fall under this category include glycolic acid, lactic acid, malic acid, tartaric acid, and citric acid.

Androgenic—Hormones, such as testosterone and andros-terone, which are affiliated with the development of mas-culine characteristics of the body. Despite this, androgenic hormones are found in males and females.

Antimicrobial—Ingredients utilized to help reduce the activities of microorganisms on the skin or body.

Antioxidant—The ability of a chemical or ingredient to counteract or block the damaging effects of free radical activity. An example is vitamin E.

Antiseptic—A chemical agent that kills or retards the growth of bacteria.

Base—The chief substance of a product or compound.

Beta Hydroxy Acids (BHAs)—These acids refine skin texture by reducing stratum corneum thickness through surface exfoliation. BHAs are excellent for use in acne products due to their ability to exfoliate excessive dead cell accumulation around the opening of the sebaceous follicle. The most recognized example in this category is salicylic acid.

Binder—Substances that hold products or compounds together. Glycerin is an example.

Bioactive or bioavailable—This refers to an ingredient that maintains its therapeutic healing properties and will work synergistically with the body's own healing mechanisms.

Blackhead—A non-inflammatory acne lesion filled with excess oil and dead skin cells. Blackheads are also referred to as "open comedones," as the surface of the skin remains open and appears darkened due to oxidation and the refraction of light from the exposed oil. (See "open comedone," below.)

Blocks—Used in skincare product formulations, blocks offer protection from the sun's ultraviolet rays by covering the skin. Thus they offer complete protection, unlike screens.

Buffer—A buffer is a compound that is added to a formulation with the intention of keeping the formulation's pH from being too low as the acid concentration is increased.

Chronological Skin Damage—This type of skin damage is due to the natural aging process. An inevitable type of skin damage, chronological aging becomes apparent in one's mid-twenties.

Closed Comedone—Commonly known as a whitehead, these are non-inflammatory comedones with a white center. (See "whitehead," below.)

Collagen—The principle proteins in connective tissues, collagen enhances the strength of the skin and improves its elasticity.

Comedo—Characterized by a plugged and, therefore, enlarged hair follicle, there are two types of comedones: closed comedones, also called "whiteheads," and open comedones, also called "blackheads."

Comedogenic—An ingredient or product that promotes the development of blockages in pilosebaceous (hair) follicles and, thus, causes the formation of comedones.

Cosmeceutical—A combination of the words cosmetic and pharmaceutical, this term is used to describe cosmetic preparations with biologically active ingredients that claim to offer medical or drug-like benefits. Most cosmeceuticals are available over-the-counter. Examples include certain anti-aging creams and moisturizers.

Depressed Scar—A type of acne scar that occurs due to the loss of tissue.

Dermabrasion—A type of cosmetic procedure whereby the outermost layer of the skin is removed via a handheld tool. Dermabrasion is effective in diminishing many types of scars, wrinkles, and age spots.

Dermis—The layer of skin between the epidermis and hypodermis. It is composed of two layers—the papillary and reticular dermis. The structural components of the dermis are collagen, elastic fibers, and extrafibrillar matrix.

Eczema—A common skin condition characterized by itchiness, redness, inflammation, and in severe cases, blisters that may ooze or crust. Eczema is a chronic condition.

Elastin—A protein present in connective tissue that has an elastic character. It allows tissues in the body to resume their shape after stretching and contracting.

Emollient—Found in product formulations, an emollient is a substance that helps to smooth and soften the skin while preventing water loss.

Emulsifying Agents—Found in product formulations, an

emulsifier is a substance that helps oil and water to mix. Common emulsifiers include carbomer and polysorbate.

Environmental Damage—This type of skin damage is that which is caused by the environmental conditions one encounters. These may include sun exposure, pollution, and smoking.

Epidermis—The outermost layer of the skin that is largely composed of keratin. Keratin acts as the skin's natural barrier to the outer environment. The epidermis is comprised of four to five layers, depending on its location on the body. These layers include (in descending order of occurrence): stratum corneum, stratum lucidum, stratum granulosum, stratum spinosum, and stratum basale.

Exfoliation—The process whereby the built-up layers of keratin are removed from the skin's surface. Exfoliation may be conducted by chemical or mechanical means.

Extrinsic Aging—The effect of outside influences on skin health. The best-known example is sun exposure.

Fair Packaging and Labeling Act—A law that requires manufacturers to follow specific criteria when developing product labels, including listing product ingredients in the order of concentration.

Follicle—A tiny shaft on the skin through which a hair grows. This is also the area where sebum is excreted from the sebaceous glands before appearing on the surface of the skin.

Free Radicals—Atoms or molecules with an unpaired electron. They damage DNA, the cellular membrane and the connective tissue components of the dermis, particularly collagen. This results in cell damage, alterations in the structure of the cell membrane, and decreased skin elasticity and pliability. Free radicals may also diminish the efficacy of the skin's immune system as they impact the Langerhans cells.

Gram Negative Folliculitis—This type of acne may develop after antiobiotics have been used for an extensive period to treat acne vulgaris. It is characterized by the presence of pustules, nodules, and cysts.

Humectant—A substance with the ability to attract water. Humectants are usually found in moisturizing lotions and creams and are used to prevent the evaporation of moisture from the skin. An example is glycerin.

Hypertrophic Scar—A type of acne scar that is raised above the skin. This type of scar is developed due to an excess of collagen, which is produced in response to the acne lesion.

Hypoallergenic—A term used to describe a cosmetic product that does not cause an allergic reaction. Because the causes and varieties of allergies are so broad, it is difficult to claim that a product is truly hypoallergenic.

Hypodermis—The innermost section of skin and the thickest of the three, the hypodermis is mainly comprised of adipose tissue (the body's fat stores).

Inflammation—The biological response of vascular tissue to harmful stimuli, including pathogens, damaged cells, or irritants. Inflammation is the body's protective attempt to remove the injurious stimuli while initiating the tissue's healing process.

International Aloe Science Council (IASC)—A nonprofit trade organization dedicated to providing the world with the highest quality of aloe. The IASC is the governing body that certifies high-quality aloe.

Intrinsic Aging—The part of the aging process that is due to the actual passing of time and hereditary factors. An example is expression lines on the face.

Keloid—A less common type of raised acne scar, keloids tend to grow beyond the original site of injury and do not diminish over time. They are more common in individuals with darker skin.

Keratin—Found in the structural matrix of cells in the epidermis, keratin is responsible for making the outer layer of skin somewhat waterproof.

Keratinocytes—Cells that produce keratin, a protein that protects the skin.

Keratosis Pilaris—A skin condition whereby keratin builds up and plugs the hair follicle, resulting in small bumps on the upper arms, thighs, and buttocks, most commonly.

Laser Skin Resurfacing—A type of cosmetic procedure whereby pulsating beams of light are used to heat the skin's dermis layer. This results in exfoliating the keratin and stimulating collagen production. It also tightens the skin by contracting collagen fibers and, thereby, reduces wrinkles and enlarged pores.

Lipids—Oily or fatty natural substances that include fats, oils, and waxes. By weight, lipids constitute 6 to 10 percent of the normal corneum layer and are essential for its healthy structure and function.

Macule—Generally flat, reddish spots that are caused by inflammatory acne lesions, macules "mark the spot" where a lesion once was and remain for six months or more. They do, however, eventually disappear, leaving no trace.

Microdermabrasion—A cosmetic procedure similar to dermabrasion but whereby only the surface cells of the skin are removed, resulting in no additional wounds.

Neutralized—A condition that is present when a chemical product is added to a formulation to bring its pH near 7, or neutral.

Nodule—A type of inflammatory acne lesion that develops after the hair follicle ruptures, nodules are large, hard lumps below the skin's surface. Nodules are often painful and take weeks to months to heal.

Nodulocystic Acne—This type of acne is characterized by the presence of numerous pus-filled cysts, most often on the face, neck, and back. It causes significant discomfort and often leads to extensive scarring.

Non-comedogenic—A product that is unlikely to cause comedones.

Open comedone—Commonly referred to as "blackheads," non-inflammatory comedones have a dark top and solid appearance. (See "blackhead," above.)

Oxidation—The result of combining oxygen with another substance.

Papule—An inflammatory comedone that resembles a small, red bump on the skin.

Parabens—Among the most utilized type of preservative, parabens have been used in skincare products for more than eighty years. They recently, however, came under scrutiny after Internet claims that they cause cancer. Despite this, no study has ever been able to prove a connection between parabens and the development of cancer.

Passive Skincare Agents—Ingredients that are functionally inactive and, therefore, won't affect the biology of the skin.

pH—A scale that is utilized to measure the acidity or alkalinity (another term for basic) of a given chemical ingredient or product. pH stands for "power (p) of the hydrogen (h) molecule," due to the element's role as a determinant of acidity or alkalinity. The pH scale ranges from 0 to 14 with a pH of 7 being neutral. A pH less than 7 is acidic while a pH greater than 7 is alkaline.

Pharmaceutical-Grade—The highest ingredient grade used in skincare products, pharmaceutical-grade ingredients are required to be 99.9% pure.

Preservative—A substance that is added to a product formulation to kill bacteria or prevent bacterial growth and to prevent spoilage. An example is methylparaben.

Propionibacterium Acnes (P. acnes)—A type of bacterium found on the skin of all adult humans, P. acnes is the bacterium that is responsible for the development of acne.

Psoriasis—A common skin condition characterized by patches of redness with flaky patches (scales). Psoriasis may cause itchiness and discomfort. It is a chronic condition.

Pustule—An inflammatory comedone that resembles a whitehead. A ring of redness may be observed around it. Pustules contain pus, which is a mixture of dead bacteria, fluids, and other waste materials.

Retinoid—A natural or synthetic substance derived from vitamin A. Retinoids help repair intrinsic damage and photo-damaged skin.

Rosacea—A skin condition characterized by patches of redness, inflammation, and spider-like blood vessels. Rosacea is a chronic condition.

Screen—Added to skincare products, a screen selectively absorbs ultraviolet light. The measurement by which sunscreens prevent ultraviolet damage is referred to as Sun Protection Factor (SPF). An example of a screen is oxybenzone.

Sebaceous glands—Attached to the hair follicles and found mostly in the face, neck, back, and chest, these glands produce an oily substance called sebum. Acne lesions have their origin in the sebaceous glands.

Sebum—The oily substance produced by the sebaceous glands.

Sodium Laureth Sulfate—A surfactant used in cleansers, sodium laureth sulfate can be irritating for those with particularly sensitive skin.

Solvent—Used in product formulations to give the product its proper consistency, a solvent is a substance that dissolves other ingredients or suspends them. Examples include alcohol and water.

Stratum Basale—The bottom layer of the epidermis.

Stratum Corneum—The top or outermost layer of the epidermis

Subcutaneous tissue (hypodermis)—The lower layer of the skin. The hypodermis consists primarily of loose connective tissues and globules of fat. It contains larger blood vessels and nerves than those found in the dermis.

Sunscreen—Specific chemicals or compounds designed to protect the skin from harmful UV rays. Sunscreens can absorb, reflect, and/or scatter the UV radiation, thereby shielding skin from the damaging effects of the sun.

Surfactants—Used in skincare product formulations, surfactants help products spread more easily and dissolve dirt and oil present on the skin. An example is sodium laureth sulfate.

Ultraviolet A (UVA)—The longest UV rays. UVA rays penetrate the dermis where they break down collagen and elastin fibrils, causing the skin to look aged. UVA only burns in large doses and is, therefore, the type of UV ray used in most tanning beds and booths.

Ultraviolet B (UVB)—The second longest UV rays. UVB rays cause most skin cancers and are responsible for sunburns. While some UVB rays penetrate the dermis, most stop at the basal layer. UVB are much stronger than UVA rays, despite the fact that UVA rays are longer and penetrate the dermis.

Viscosity—The degree of density, thickness, stickiness, and adhesiveness of a substance. It also refers to the resistance of a substance to change form and the resistance of a substance to flow.

Whitehead—An acne lesion that forms when oil and skin cells block the opening of a hair follicle, hence their alternative name of "closed comedones." Whiteheads are covered by a thin layer of skin cells, which allows them to reflect light—hence their white color. (See "closed comedone," above.)

SOURCES

1. Mintel. "Anti-aging Skincare (U.S.)." March, 2009.

2. Muise, A. and S. Desmarais. "Women's Perceptions and Use of 'Anti-Aging' Products." *Sex Roles,* 63, *no.1–2* (2010): 126–137.

3. Chung, HY, HJ Kim, JW Kim, and BP Yu. "The Inflammation Hypothesis of Aging." *Annals of the New York Academy of Sciences,* 928, (April 2001): 327–335.

4. Beckman, KB and BN Ames. "The Free Radical Theory of Aging Matures." *Physiological Reviews,* 78, *no.2* (April 1, 1998): 547–581.

5. Grazul-Bilska, AT, JJ Bilski, DA Redmer, LP Reynolds, KM Abdullah, and A. Abdullah. "Antioxidant Capacity of 3D

Human Skin EpiDerm™ Model: Effects of Skin Moisturizers." *International Journal of Cosmetic Science*, 31, *no*.3 (June 2009): 201–208.

6. Purba, M., A. Kouris-Blazos, N. Wattanapenpaiboon, et al. "Skin Wrinkling: Can Food Make a Difference?" *Journal of the American College of Nutrition*, 20, *no*.1 (February 2001): 71–80.

7. Cosgrove M, O. Franco, S. Granger, et al. "Dietary Nutrient Intakes and Skin-aging Appearance Among Middle-aged American Women." *American Journal of Clinical Nutrition*, 86, *no*.4 (October 2007): 1225–1231.

8. Darbre, PD, A. Aljarrah, WR Miller, NR Coldham, MJ Sauer, and GS Pope. "Concentrations of Parabens in Human Breast Tumours." *Journal of Applied Toxicology*, 24, *no*.1 (2004): 5–13.

9. Macias, CA, MV Kameneva, JJ Tenhunen, JC Puyana, and MP Fink. "Survival in A Rat Model of Lethal Hemorrhagic Shock Is Prolonged Following Resuscitation With A Small Volume of A Solution Containing A Drag-Reducing Polymer Derived From Aloe Vera." *Shock*, 22, *no*.2 (August 2004): 151–156.

10. Abdullah, A, KM Abdullah, AT Grazul-Bilska, ML Johnson, JJ Bilski, DA Redmer, and LP Reynolds. "Wound Healing: the Role of Growth Factors." *Drugs of Today*, 39, *no.*10 (2003): 787–800.

11. Abdullah, KM, A. Abdullah, ML Johnson, JJ Bilski, K. Petry, DA Redmer, LP Reynolds, and AT Grazul-Bilska. "Effects of Aloe Vera on Gap Junctional Intercellular Communication and Proliferation of Human Diabetic and Nondiabetic Skin Fibroblasts." *Journal of Alternative and Complementary Medicine.* 9, *no.*5 (October 2003): 711–718.

12. Mitsuishi, T, T. Shimoda, Y. Mitsui, Y. Kuriyama, and S. Kawana. "The Effects of Topical Application of Phytonadione, Retinol and Vitamins C and E on Infraorbital Dark Circles and Wrinkles of the Lower Eyelids." *Journal of Cosmetic Dermatology.* 3, *no.*2 (April 2004): 73–75.

13. American Academy of Dermatology. "Acne." Updated November 2009. http://www.aad.org/public/publications/pamphlets/common_acne.html.

14. Gollnick, H, W. Cunliffe, D. Berson, B. Derno, A. Finlay, JJ Leyden, AR Shalita, and D. Thiboutot. "Management of Acne: A Report From a Global Alliance to Improve

Outcomes in Acne." Supplement, *Journal of the American Academy of Dermatology*, 49, no.1 (July 2003): S1–37.

15. Jancin, B. "Teens With Acne Cite Shame, Embarrassment About Skin." *Skin & Allergy News* (January 2004): 28.

16. Adebamowo, CA, D. Spiegelman, FW Danby, AL Frazier, WC Willett, MD Holmes. "High School Dietary Dairy Intake and Teenage Acne." *Journal of the American Academy of Dermatology*, 52, no.2 (February 2005): 207–14.

17. Dupree, LC. "Evaluating the Link Between Diet and Acne." *U.S. Pharmacist*, 34, no.4 (July 2009): 26–37

18. Green, Orchard, Cerio, et al. "A Clinicopathological Study of the Effects of Topical Retinyl Propionate Cream in Skin Photoaging." *Clinical and Experimental Dermotology*, 23, no.4 (July 1998): 162–167.

19. Wang, CM, CL Huang, CTS Hu, and HL Chan. "The Effect of Glycolic Acid on the Treatment of Acne is Asian Skin." *Dermatologic Surgery*, 23, no.1 (January 1997): 23–29.

20. Zander, E. and S. Weisman. "Treatment of Acne Vulgaris With Salicylic Acid Pads." *Clinical Therapeutics*, 14, no.2 (March-April 1992): 247–53.

21. Breneman, DL and MC Ariano. "Successful Treatment of Acne Vulgaris in Women With a New Topical Sodium Sulfacetamide/Sulfur Lotion." *International Journal of Dermatology*, 32, *no.*5 (May 1993): 365–7.

22. Takahasi, T, R. Kokubo, and M. Sakaino. "Antimicrobial Activities of Eucalyptus Leaf Extracts and Flavonoids from *Eucalyptus maculata*." *Letters in Applied Microbiology*, 39, *no.*1 (July 2004): 60–64.

23. Bassett, IB, DL Pannowitz, RS Barnetson. "A Comparative Study of Tea-Tree Oil Versus Benzoyl Peroxide in the Treatment of Acne." *Medical Journal of Australia*, 153, *no.*8 (1990): 455–8.

24. Porock, D, S. Nikoletti, L. Kristjanson. "Management of Radiation Skin Reactions: Literature Review and Clinical Application." *Plastic Surgical Nursing*, 19, *no.*4 (1999): 185–92, 223.

25. Lissoni, P, F. Rovelli, F. Brivio, R. Zago, M. Colciago, G. Messina, A. Mora, and G. Porro. "A Randomized Study of Chemotherapy Versus Biochemotherapy with Chemotherapy Plus *Aloe arborescens* in Patients with Metastatic Cancer." *In Vivo*, 23, *no.*1 (January-February 2009): 171–5.

ABOUT THE AUTHOR

Dr. Ahmed Abdullah is a board-certified plastic surgeon and a recognized expert on the restorative and medicinal effects of aloe vera. Additionally, he is an associate clinical professor in plastic surgery at the University of North Dakota School of Medicine, and founder/formulator of the Lexli line of aloe-based professional skincare.

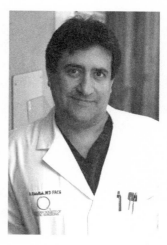

Despite his expertise in plastic surgery, Dr. Abdullah has proven that many common skin concerns can be avoided by optimizing skin health. His research has shown that the use of pharmaceutical-grade aloe vera is a beneficial tool in that effort. Thus, Dr. Abdullah travels the world educating licensed skincare professionals and consumers alike about the proper ways to utilize aloe in skincare applications, the essential steps to ensuring the skin's basic needs are met, and setting the record straight on prevalent skincare myths. Furthermore, he still sees patients regularly at his practices in Fargo, North Dakota and Dubai, United Arab Emirates.

A member of the International Aloe Science Council (IASC), Dr. Abdullah has served on its board of directors. Furthermore, he is a diplomat of the American Board of Surgery and the American Board of Plastic Surgery, and serves on the Ethics Committee of the North Dakota Medical Association.

Dr. Abdullah earned his medical degree from Northwestern University in Chicago and completed his residency at the University of Texas Medical Branch in Galveston, Texas. He is married to Dr. Kay Abdullah, a board-certified surgeon, with whom he has twin sons—Alex and Ali.